Black Women's Risk
for HIV
Rough Living

Haworth Psychosocial Issues of HIV/AIDS
R. Dennis Shelby, PhD
Editor

HIV and Social Work: A Practitioner's Guide edited by David M. Aronstein and Bruce J. Thompson

HIV/AIDS and the Drug Culture: Shattered Lives by Elizabeth Hagan and Joan Gormley

AIDS and Mental Health Practice: Clinical and Policy Issues edited by Michael Shernoff

AIDS and Development in Africa: A Social Science Perspective by Kempe Ronald Hope Sr.

Women's Experiences with HIV/AIDS: Mending Fractured Selves by Desirée Ciambrone

Hotel Ritz—Comparing Mexican and U.S. Street Prostitutes: Factors in HIV/AIDS Transmission by David J. Bellis

Practice Issues in HIV/AIDS Services: Empowerment-Based Models and Program Applications edited by Ronald J. Mancoske and James Donald Smith

Preventing AIDS: Community-Science Collaborations edited by Benjamin P. Bowser, Shiraz I. Mishra, Cathy J. Reback, and George F. Lemp

Couples of Mixed HIV Status: Clinical Issues and Interventions by Nancy L. Beckerman

Lesbian Women and Sexual Health: The Social Construction of Risk and Susceptibility by Kathleen A. Dolan

Behind the Eight Ball: Sex for Crack Cocaine Exchange and Poor Black Women by Tanya Telfair Sharpe

HIV, Substance Abuse, and Communication Disorders in Children by Robert Martin Screen and Dorian Lee-Wilkerson

Black Women's Risk for HIV: Rough Living by Quinn M. Gentry

Black Women's Risk for HIV
for HIV
Rough Living

Quinn M. Gentry, MBA, PhD

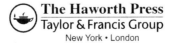
The Haworth Press
Taylor & Francis Group
New York • London

For more information on this book or to order, visit
http://www.haworthpress.com/store/product.asp?sku=5784

or call 1-800-HAWORTH (800-429-6784) in the United States and Canada
or (607) 722-5857 outside the United States and Canada

or contact orders@HaworthPress.com

The Haworth Press, Taylor & Francis Group, 270 Madison Avenue, New York, NY 10016.

PUBLISHER'S NOTE
The development, preparation, and publication of this work has been undertaken with great care. However, the Publisher, employees, editors, and agents of The Haworth Press are not responsible for any errors contained herein or for consequences that may ensue from use of materials or information contained in this work. The Haworth Press is committed to the dissemination of ideas and information according to the highest standards of intellectual freedom and the free exchange of ideas. Statements made and opinions expressed in this publication do not necessarily reflect the views of the Publisher, Directors, management, or staff of The Haworth Press, or an endorsement by them.

Identities and circumstances of individuals discussed in this book have been changed to protect confidentiality.

Cover design by Marylouise Doyle.

Library of Congress Cataloging-in-Publication Data

Gentry, Quinn M.
     Black women's risk for HIV : Rough living / Quinn M. Gentry.
        p. ; cm.
     Includes bibliographical references and index.
     ISBN: 978-0-7890-3169-3 (hard : alk. paper)
     ISBN: 978-0-7890-3170-9 (soft : alk. paper)
     1. AIDS (Disease) in women—Risk factors—Georgia—Atlanta. 2. AIDS (Disease) in women—Social aspects—Georgia—Atlanta. 3. HIV infections—Risk factors—Georgia—Atlanta. 4. HIV infections—Social aspects—Georgia—Atlanta. 5. African American women—Health and hygiene—Georgia—Atlanta. 6. African American women—Diseases—Georgia—Atlanta. 7. African American women—Georgia—Atlanta—Social conditions. 8. Atlanta (Georgia)—Social conditions. I. Title.
     [DNLM: 1. HIV Infections—ethnology—Georgia. 2. African Americans—Georgia. 3. Risk Factors—Georgia. 4. Socioeconomic Factors—Georgia. 5. Women's Health—Georgia. WC 503.4 AG4 G339b 2007]

     RA643.84.G46G46 2007
     362.196'97920082—dc22

                                                                                        2007026487

In loving memory of
Irene Ferguson (1910-1981), my maternal grandmother

In loving reflection of
the African-American women who have guided and nurtured
me through the years. You were my first black feminist
teachers and your examples by living lives of survival against
seemingly insurmountable odds are by far greater than
any other intellectual or theoretical lessons.

A special thanks to the women in the Rough who granted me
access to their lives. One in particular trusted me enough to make
me a part of her "change team" and I am forever grateful.

A special dedication to Henry for the way you stepped up to the
challenge of loving, learning, and leading me through some
"Rough" times of my own. Together we can do all things
because we are strong through Christ who strengthens us.

Finally, this book is written under the mentoring of my mother
and other mothers in my life including my birth mother
(Clara), my godmother (Lillian "Matoo"), my aunts (Inez, Mary,
Pauline, Mattie, and Leannia), and my community mothers
(Mrs. Sanford, Mrs. Washburn, Ms. Lane, Mrs. Manner,
Mrs. Ammons, Ms. Duncan, Mrs. Bentley-Grier, Dr. Buggs,
Rachel Alexander, Rita Culver, and Betty Smith). Your guiding
principles at key points in my life were extremely significant
in shaping me to be the woman I am today.

ABOUT THE AUTHOR

Quinn Gentry, PhD, is an Atlanta-based behavior scientist and clinical researcher whose work focuses on high-risk youth development, women's substance abuse and mental health, and community-based systems of care. Dr. Gentry currently is a principal investigator for several social and health projects for Messages of Empowerment Productions, LLC—a minority and woman-owned firm specializing in program evaluation and behavior interventions for high-risk populations. She also is a National Institute of Health-sponsored clinical researcher where she is developing organizational and evaluation capacity for AID Atlanta's HIV-prevention services and programs, and she has teaching appointments at Emory University and Georgia State University. A licensed minister and national speaker, Dr. Gentry is leading the efforts for a faith-based substance abuse recovery program titled, "Recover Me"; and an intervention for high-risk girls titled "GEMS-Girls Empowered and Motivated to Succeed." She also has developed a women's-centered empowerment program titled, "The Heart of the Matter." In addition, Dr. Gentry wrote, produced, and directed a stage play based on her clinical research with women at risk for HIV titled *Divine Intervention.*

CONTENTS

Foreword   xi
Kirk W. Elifson
Claire E. Sterk

Preface   xv

Acknowledgments   xix

Chapter 1. Introduction: This Is the Rough!   1
The Rough As a High-Risk Environment   1
Facing My Own Rough Reality   5
Background of the Health Intervention Project   8
Ethnographic Research Methods   10
Theoretical Framework   15
Research Objectives   22

Chapter 2. Living in the Rough   25
Street Women   26
House Women   46
Principles to Guide HIV Prevention Initiatives Based
   on Women's Living Arrangements   60

Chapter 3. Rough Family Relations   63
Growing Up Decent   66
Growing Up Street   77
Making Sense of Decent and Street Upbringing   83
Accounts of Interactions with Families of Orientation   84
Deceiving Family Members   90
Engaging in Frequent Interaction with Family   91
Principles to Guide Family-Focused
   HIV Prevention Initiatives   94

Chapter 4. Intimate Relationships in the Rough   97
Overview of the Five Stages of Intimate Partner
   Relationships   99

The Courtship Stage 100
The Commitment Stage 103
The Conflict Stage 112
The Compromise Stage 115
The Conclusion Stage 120
Principles to Guide a Couples-Centered HIV Prevention
 Initiative 126

Chapter 5. Mothering in the Rough **133**
Maintaining Custody on the Margin 136
Giving Up Temporary Custody to Kin 140
Disclosing Drug Use to Authorities 146
Grandmothering As a Hopeful Experience 147
Hopeless Mothers Themes 148
Cycling Between Hopeless and Hopeful Mothering 159
Principles to Guide Addressing Issues Related
 to Motherhood As HIV Prevention Initiatives 164

**Chapter 6. When Work and Welfare Disappear
in the Rough** **167**
Hustling Knowledge 169
Renting Space 180
Shoplifting 182
Odd-Job Hustlers 184
Principles to Guide Economic-Focused HIV Prevention
 Initiatives 190

Chapter 7. Religiosity in the Rough **195**
The Churched 196
The Unchurched 201
A Theoretical Framework for Understanding Potential
 Roles for Inner-City Churches in HIV Prevention 204
Principles to Guide Faith-Based HIV Prevention Initiatives 205

Chapter 8. Reducing Risk in the Rough **211**
Leaving the Rough for Drug Treatment 212
Practicing Safer Sex 221
Making Other Changes 224
Making No Changes in Behavior 228

**Chapter 9. Black Feminist Theory As Behavior Change
Theory and Practice**   **233**
Rethinking the HIP Intervention   241
An HIV Prevention Model for Black Women Guided
by Black Feminism   245

References   **249**

Index   **257**

NOTES FOR PROFESSIONAL LIBRARIANS
AND LIBRARY USERS

This is an original book title published by The Haworth Press, Taylor & Francis Group. Unless otherwise noted in specific chapters with attribution, materials in this book have not been previously published elsewhere in any format or language.

CONSERVATION AND PRESERVATION NOTES

All books published by The Haworth Press and its imprints are printed on certified pH neutral, acid-free book grade paper. This paper meets the minimum requirements of American National Standard for Information Sciences-Permanence of Paper for Printed Material, ANSI Z39.48-1984.

DIGITAL OBJECT IDENTIFIER (DOI) LINKING

The Haworth Press is participating in reference linking for elements of our original books. (For more information on reference linking initiatives, please consult the CrossRef Web site at www.crossref.org.) When citing an element of this book such as a chapter, include the element's Digital Object Identifier (DOI) as the last item of the reference. A Digital Object Identifier is a persistent, authoritative, and unique identifier that a publisher assigns to each element of a book. Because of its persistence, DOIs will enable The Haworth Press and other publishers to link to the element referenced, and the link will not break over time. This will be a great resource in scholarly research.

Foreword

Around the same time that many believed that no infectious disease was going to challenge medical sciences biomedical advances, the HIV/AIDS epidemic emerged. Challenges arose, as it turned out to be difficult to identify the constantly mutating virus that causes HIV/AIDS, as well the variety of signs and symptoms that make up the syndrome. During the early 1980s, a test to identify infection with the human immunodeficiency virus (HIV) was developed. The expectation was that a cure would soon follow. However, finding a cure has proven to be much more difficult, and well into the third decade of the HIV/AIDS epidemic, no effective vaccine has been identified. The furthest we have come is to have treatments that slow the progression of the disease, thereby changing it to a chronic condition.

Initially, HIV/AIDS was largely viewed as a syndrome that impacted select populations. Among these were men who engaged in sex with other men and users of illicit drugs. These so-called risk groups involved human beings who already faced stigmatization in society. However, as it became clear that not all members of a specific risk group became infected, the language shifted to risk behaviors. Whereas this may be perceived as a positive trend, it also resulted in blaming those who became infected for their status. Exceptions were made for those individuals who belong to risk groups, such as persons who became infected through a blood transfusion or persons who were engaged in mainstream sexual relationships and whose partner caused them to acquire the virus. Interestingly, the notion of risk behavior and the associated blaming did not apply to them.

As we have entered the twenty-first century, a common route of HIV transmission is through unsafe heterosexual contact. Among those who became infected through unsafe sex, an overwhelming majority are women. Moreover, they tend to be women of color who reside in

Black Women's Risk for HIV: Rough Living
© 2007 by The Haworth Press, Taylor & Francis Group. All rights reserved.
doi:10.1300/5784_a

poor inner-city neighborhoods in metropolitan areas across the southeastern United States. Whereas the Centers for Disease Control and Prevention and other agencies have been reporting on this trend for close to a decade, few initiatives have resulted in effectively curtailing the spread of HIV among such women. As Gentry points out, those women most impacted by the HIV/AIDS epidemic tend to be black and poor, and they have limited resources. She describes how gender, race, and class intersect but also how few risk reduction interventions have taken this reality into consideration.

Gentry's monograph focuses on African-American women who reside in the Rough, a typical inner-city neighborhood like so many others in the United States. Once a supportive community, the members of which were actively engaged in the Civil Rights Movement, the Rough has become a community lacking in social capital. It is characterized by a crumbling physical and social infrastructure. The Rough became the site of a community-based HIV risk reduction intervention targeting African-American women who used illicit drugs, specifically those who smoked crack cocaine or those who injected drugs such as heroin or cocaine. This became known as the Health Intervention Project (HIP). Working toward her doctoral degree in sociology, after having utilized her MBA degree in the business world, Gentry was eager to apply her newly acquired theoretical and methodological knowledge. This monograph is an extraordinary high-quality product to emerge from her dissertation research. Initially, she became one of the HIP intervention specialists and interviewers. She describes how two weeks into the project she recognized one of the HIP women as a former eighth-grade classmate. This motivated her further to understand what was happening, and more important, to learn what needed to be done.

Gentry brings years of personal experience, extensive knowledge, and excellent research skills to this monograph. In *Black Women's Risk for HIV: Rough Living* she reveals an outstanding sociological imagination. She does not shy away from applying her sociological insights to "real life." Based on her ethnographic inquiry that included participant observation, mapping, and interviewing that is guided by a black feminist perspective, she presents a paradigm for HIV risk reduction that is grounded in the women's perspective. In doing so she highlights the importance of considering the historical journey of African-American women in the United States, including the role of the church and the women's approach to religiosity and spirituality. She specifically highlights the importance of agency among African-American women, a perspective that often is ignored and a trait seldom associated with disempowered and poor women. In doing so, Gentry also recognizes the complex set of social roles most women typically occupy, including the associated role strain. For example, she explores women's roles as family members and the impact of the family of origin on their current functioning as well as its role in terms of social support. Next, she highlights the women's roles, such as being a partner in an intimate relationship and being a mother. By recognizing the women's agency and their social roles, HIV risk reduction interventions need to build on the existing agency and provide advocacy. In addition, such interventions may gain from including family members and partners. This approach also links the women's individual circumstances to the larger social context, including the community in which they reside and its characteristics as well as structural and policy influences. Gentry takes a refreshing look at the phenomenon of the devastating impact of the HIV/AIDS epidemic on poor African-American women. She challenges our assumptions about the women's lives, including the presumed reasons for their weak positions and our biases in terms of their potential for a brighter future. This book is a treasure for scholars in disciplines such as sociology, anthropology, psychology, and public health as well as for social and health service providers and policy makers.

Kirk W. Elifson
Georgia State University

Claire E. Sterk
Emory University

Preface

I started my journey into the Rough—part activist and part scholar—to make a difference in the lives of women at high risk for HIV. But somewhere along the way, each client made a difference in my life because I was open to learning about ways in which our lives were similar. These women were at risk for HIV mainly because of substance abuse, and I recalled the first time that I even heard the words HIV/AIDS and crack cocaine as an inner-city adolescent. I am not HIV positive and have never smoked crack cocaine, but these two social and health epidemics are very much a part of my personal history. Every woman I worked with caused me to reexamine my own behavior and come to accept that, although my outcomes were different, my environment and experiences were similar to many of the women at risk for HIV. What I learned through these discussions is that black women are talking tough but living rough—living rough in terms of trying to make sense of love and intimate relationships as grounded in trust and honesty. Yet we are told to begin our love relationships by confronting our potential soul mates with discussions about condom use and HIV/AIDS status. In public we say we are doing just that. However, the statistical data about the spread of HIV among black women tell a different story about our private lives. We are talking tough about our high standards for a good man, but our pool of eligible bachelors has become a cesspool of black men who are disproportionately either in prison, on parole, or probation. So we talk tough about safe sex in theory, but our practice is rough and often leads to risky behavior—behavior we are reluctant to admit for fear of being judged as promiscuous, having low self-esteem, or simply not being careful enough in the choices we make.

I can relate to the mixed messages that drive black women to talk tough and live rough. Throughout my childhood, I remember hearing in church and school that I was special, unique, different, gifted,

Black Women's Risk for HIV: Rough Living
© 2007 by The Haworth Press, Taylor & Francis Group. All rights reserved.
doi:10.1300/5784_b

smart, and destined for greatness. At the same time, the messages from my family were that "you're no better than anybody else," "you argue too much," "you talk too much," "you're too loud and too fast." Hearing what I thought were conflicting messages caused me to be confused about who I was and what was expected of me as a poor black girl transitioning into womanhood.

When I returned to the Rough some twenty years after growing up in a rough-like neighborhood, the women in the Rough helped clarify the ways in which both sets of messages from my socializing agents could co-exist. Messages that I was unique sent me searching for ways in which my life and experiences were different from the women I worked with as part of this clinical intervention. But messages from my family that I was no better than anybody else humbled me to look for ways in which my everyday life, past and present, was like that of the women in my study. I could not imagine how my life would be different or similar to the women in this book who had family, church, school, and community which had failed them in their childhood. Like some of the women in the book, my life started out in dire poverty; unlike many of them, I was socially secure with a stay-at-home grandmother who, with only a fourth-grade education, taught me to read and write at the age of 3. Like many of these women, I have compromised my self-worth in search of intimate love; unlike many of them, no intimate partner ever offered me crack cocaine. In my senior year I was a valedictorian destined for college, a participant in church activities, voted best all-around student by the faculty and most likely to succeed by the senior class; with scholarships waiting for me at several top-ranked colleges and having heard the Nancy Reagan slogan of "just say no"—I still said "yes" to my drug-dealing boyfriend when he said "here, smoke this joint." I can only imagine what my life would be like today had that been a good experience. As it turns out, I just didn't get it. My two good girlfriends growing up tried to get me to drink wine coolers, but my stomach ached to the point that again I just didn't get it. So it wasn't that I didn't try alcohol and drugs or unprotected sex, I just didn't get caught up. Choosing to believe the messages that I am special may have resulted in a self-fulfilling prophecy over time, but it did not guarantee that I would not give in to high-risk behavior. However, when I challenge other "mainstream" women to rethink their past and present risk factors for HIV, many choose to lie, deny, or clarify why their lives are nothing like my clients' lives. Paradoxically, their choice to remain silent or not search for common ground actually increases their chances of becoming infected.

The women whose lives are represented in this book highlight the need for us to redefine ourselves as empowered black women—women with high levels of self-esteem and self-worth that give us the courage to tell the truth about our lives and how rough it really is to navigate love and relationships. We have heard for years that the faces of HIV/AIDS have changed, but we fail to consider that the factors leading to risk are as different as the diverse faces. Just as the faces and factors have shifted, so too has the blame. We blame the continued spread of HIV/AIDS in the black community on those with the least resources and power to fight back individually and structurally: poor black girls and women.

Since completing this book, I have embarked upon a fight of my own—that of helping black women who do not smoke crack understand that our risk factors are entangled with those of our sisters with fewer resources. As long as we are looking for love in the same places, our lives are forever interrelated. Hence this book is grounded in my belief that I should share what I have learned about direct and indirect risks for HIV. As I continue to look for ways to combine activism with scholarship, this book is merely a stop along the journey of learning how to tell black women's truth in a way that produces knowledge about us from us, raises our consciousness about issues affecting all black women's lives, and empowers us to act against anything that affects some of us directly and others of us indirectly. Until all black women have voice, I am my sister's speaker. And I speak the truth about black women's risk for HIV.

Acknowledgments

First, I give honor to God who is the head of my life for giving me the gifts needed to think critically, write creatively, and act compassionately on behalf of women who are indeed within our reach. To my soul mate, Henry Gentry, I say thank you for being that inspiration in the midnight hour, coaching me to victory in all that I attempt. You came in and pushed me to "step up in there." You are the greatest! I would like to thank my Elizabeth Baptist Church family and my Women's Institute of Ministry sisters, as you provided the spiritual energy and nurturing needed throughout this endeavor. I am particularly grateful for my Master Life Group, the Couples' Ministry, and my Friday Night Bible Study Posse. In addition, I thank my sister friends Michelle, Syreeta, Neena, Joanne, Chelsea, Lucy, Sarita, and Kijua. Also, my Coalition of 100 Black Women, Metro Atlanta Chapter, are phenomenal women, whose collective accomplishments and achievements helped me visualize the possibilities of my own success as an author, lecturer, and activist. Finally, to my longest and dearest friend, Tyronda: we have a special bond, as we know the Rough all too well from our personal plights, but by the grace of God we are miracles, and I am so glad God granted me the privilege of calling you sister.

Dr. Kirk Elifson! What can I say? You took a diamond in the "Rough" who had only energy and passion and set her on the path of "scholar." Your encouragement has made the difference in my merging "intellectual activism." Dr. Claire Sterk, as an emerging black feminist activist and scholar, I cling to your every word, suggestion, idea, and even your mannerisms. I am now a carrier of the "lineless book," which serves as a constant reminder that real ethnographers are always watching and recording. You have modeled the way by lifting as you climb. In searching for my own identity as an insider activist,

I didn't have to look far for a successful role model. Thank you all for your patience and guidance, and for never being too busy to mentor. Many thanks also to the individuals who are serving and acting on behalf of individuals affected and infected by HIV/AIDS and drug abuse at AID Atlanta, Positive Impact, Another Chance, St. Jude's Recovery Center, and Mary Hall Freedom House.

In addition to these very dedicated individuals, I would like to thank the entire Sociology department at Georgia State University for the wealth of knowledge and genuine interest in my academic career. Dr. Ghamari, you are the best black feminist scholar I know. Thank you for a great unorthodox story to tell my children about my experiences as a graduate student. Dr. Denise Donnelly, I sincerely appreciate your diligence in helping me make sense of family and gender studies. Your oral history project prompted my inquiry into the past lives of my study participants, where I discovered so much more rich detail. Dr. Ralph LaRossa, you sparked my love for qualitative research methods and I now have weekly "coding parties." Dr. Charles Jaret, your urban research ethnography project resulted in my expanding the breadth of my participant observation into "the midnight hour." The "Rough" looks totally different when the HIP House is closed. I would also like to thank the HIP House staff for your acceptance of me on the team and your dedication to the women we all grew to support. As I have dedicated this book in part to the women who entrusted their life stories to me, I express a world of gratitude to you and will honor your honesty by continuing to speak the truth about who you are, what you have experienced, and what you are capable of individually and collectively as I spread messages of empowerment to women and girls who have been interrupted with unnecessary roughness. Finally, to my mentees, in the spirit of Harriet Tubman, I have left footprints and stations along the railroad; you must walk the walk. Don't worry; I am here to guide the way!

Chapter 1

Introduction: This Is the Rough!

> I don't think anything going to be able to happen to change the situation in this community because it's just the way it is. This how this particular part runs. It's going to be like this from now on. This is the Rough!
>
> Punkin, a 25-year-old HIV-positive crack cocaine user
> and seller, sex worker, and mother of two

THE ROUGH AS A HIGH-RISK ENVIRONMENT

Punkin is a 25-year-old crack-addicted and HIV-positive sex worker who arrived in the Rough in the early 1990s as a high-risk adolescent fully engaged in the sex and drug behavior that ultimately led to her being infected with human immunodeficiency virus (HIV). By the time Punkin arrived in the Rough, long gone were the images and symbols of the neighborhood as one in which middle-class black families raised successful children, ran profitable businesses, and participated in the desegregation movement, as many of the civil rights leaders lived in and around the Rough. The Rough that Punkin came to know in the early 1990s consisted disproportionately of poor, law-abiding residents lacking resources for upward mobility. Others who remained in the Rough included the elderly and two generations of crack users and sellers. Moreover, many houses that were vacated by the upwardly mobile in the late 1970s and early 1980s evolved over time into abandoned houses and ultimately became known as crack houses. Still,

Black Women's Risk for HIV: Rough Living
© 2007 by The Haworth Press, Taylor & Francis Group. All rights reserved.
doi:10.1300/5784_01

there remain the boarded-up buildings, schools, apartments, businesses, and churches that provide evidence that at one time the Rough consisted of black families living relatively decent lives raising relatively decent children. Punkin's assertion that the Rough will not change from being characterized as a high-risk community is based on the fact that the Rough has served as the hub for chronic drug users and sellers for generations. Even in the midst of middle-class families, a few concentrated blocks of the Rough have always been infamous as an illegal drug supermarket corridor. Before the onset of crack cocaine, however, decent families dominated the Rough and held the hard-core drug sellers and chronic drug users to a few blocks of operation. In fact, because of the Rough's close proximity to the Atlanta University Center (made up of five historically black colleges and universities), it was not uncommon, prior to desegregation, to find black lawyers, professors, doctors, nurses, teachers, and clergy literally living next door to factory workers, janitors, maids, and cooks.

After the civil rights movement's major victory of desegregation, many upwardly mobile black families took flight to the suburbs, leaving the Rough with limited community leadership and role models, and over time left those remaining African Americans more isolated and devoid of formal and informal infrastructures (Massey and Denton, 1993; Staples, 1999). As there were limited efforts to restore the infrastructure, economic opportunities lessened and the socialization of children and young adults was seriously disrupted. According to Wallace (1993), "This [diminished socioeconomic opportunities] interacts with drug dependency, multiple sexual partner activity, poor access to service and resources, wider social discrimination and a palpable lack of political power to make such neighborhoods vulnerable to the rapid spread of HIV." Wallace's theory of the relationship between disintegrated neighborhoods and the spread of HIV is applicable to the Rough. The women who grew up in or near the Rough, in particular, express a deep concern that the Rough has become more fragmented and disenfranchised over time. Today the Rough suffers from chronic drug use and unemployment, as well as soaring cases of HIV/AIDS (acquired immune deficiency syndrome), destruction of housing in the poorest areas, and high concentrations of homelessness. Moreover, the demise in infrastructure has resulted in limited community-based social services in the Rough to respond to the HIV/AIDS dilemma.

As I started to make some sense of how the Rough was one of many urban neighborhoods where HIV/AIDS is taking a toll among African-American women, I wanted to have a better understanding of structural conditions that contribute to the continued spread of HIV. While a comprehensive macro perspective on the social conditions of the Rough is beyond the scope of this book, I believe it is important to highlight some of the structural forces that exist and shape the Rough as a high-risk environment. According to the U.S. Census Bureau (1990), the Rough is a "ghetto poor" neighborhood because more than 40 percent of its largely African-American residents live below the poverty line. In fact, census tract level data revealed that in the 1980s the Rough had a poverty rate of 79 percent among a population that is 97 percent African American. Some ten years later, the 2000 U.S. Census Bureau, reporting on U.S. trends in the 1990s, revealed that the poverty line for the Rough was reduced to 41 percent. Clearly this is due to a number of social and economic policies aimed at eliminating concentrated poverty in inner cities throughout America. In fact, rather than uplift the poor, social policymakers opted instead to uproot the poor. Social policies such as welfare reform and the deconstruction of public housing in exchange for mixed income developments in fact resulted in lower rates of poverty in the Rough. However, without concerted and deliberate efforts to track the paths and socioeconomic outcomes of families and inviduals leaving the Rough, social policy analysts are unable to successfully conclude that social and economic policies actually reduced the number of individuals classified as ghetto poor. But rather, through the phenomenon of gentrification, what we do know is that the number of middle class and white individuals living near the Rough increased from 1990 to 2000 in ways that would result in lower percentages of people living in poverty.

The urgency of addressing black women's risk for HIV is rooted in the devastating consequences of social and economic policies that ultimately led to the black feminzation of poverty. This phenomenon sent poor black women scrambling for economic and social survival, resulting in heightened risks for HIV infection. To put it bluntly, the black feminization of poverty is a phenomenon in which mainstream

America directly and indirectly supports policies to push black women off welfare, put them out of public housing, and place their children in foster care. At the same time, black women are becoming poorer and more desperate to maintain on the socioeconomic margins, and there is a steady rise of new cases of HIV among black women.

Today, the black feminization of poverty manifests as a key factor explaining why black women are experiencing unprecedented new cases of HIV. Recent CDC (2005) data show that HIV/AIDS is now the leading cause of death among younger African Americans, who are between the ages of 24 and 35 and at higher risks for heterosexual HIV transmission. Closely related, HIV/AIDS is the third leading cause of death for black women between the ages of 35 and 44; and the fourth leading cause of death for black women between the ages of 45 and 54. As it is clear that black women are at risk for HIV over the life course, it is extremely important that researchers move black women from the margin to the center as it relates to implementing prevention intervention programs.

By the time the HIV prevention program known as HIP (Health Intervention Project) was implemented in the Rough, this program proved too little, too limited, and too late to help Punkin, as she was already HIV positive when I met her. But for many other high-risk women, they demonstrated that despite seemingly insurmountable odds, it is possible to change one's high-risk behavior in Rough-like environments. Punkin's story, however, highlights how the lines of personal responsibility and public accountability are blurred as it relates to how high-risk children are left behind socially, economically, mentally, and educationally. Just as in Punkin's case, once high-risk and socioeconomically disadvantaged youth transition into adulthood, blame subtly shifts from the structural constraints to individual choices, as it becomes easier to blame adult women for their own troubles. Perhaps Punkin's own sociological imagination is guiding her thinking as she provides an honest and scathing critique of the Rough when she declares that nothing can be done to change a Rough-like community. As I pondered Punkin's pessimistic perspective, I began to think of how one eats the proverbial elephant—and that is one bite at a time. In this way, changing the Rough may be a larger undertaking requiring additional capacity building at multiple levels among diverse stakeholders. In the interim, however, we can change one life at a time by working intensely with high-risk women before they approach Punkin's plight of being crack addicted, HIV positive, and serving as sex workers in a high-risk community. While changing the Rough may be beyond the scope of most HIV prevention interventions, I do believe that by changing individual high-risk women's behavior, we have taken the first bite in changing the structure of the Rough.

FACING MY OWN ROUGH REALITY

I remember the day that my experiences became real and surreal in a way that intensified my personal and professional commitment to HIV prevention education and research. Less than two weeks into my applied research position on the study, I was pulling client files in preparation for the scheduled HIV prevention interventions. My heart dropped as I came across the name of one of my high school classmates who was a formal client of the program. Having grown up myself in a Rough-like neighborhood less than two miles from the Rough, it did not surprise me that I would discover I knew some of the clients. However, I was not prepared for the client file I came across belonging to a fellow honor student. I was sure it would have been the file of one of the girls from our high school who either dated drug dealers or had one or even two children upon graduation, or who had dropped out of high school altogether before our class graduated in 1986 during the heart of the "New Jack City" era. In essence, I would have predicted that the HIV prevention intervention client file I discovered would belong to a girl at the bottom of our class, or even to one who had been unengaged in extracurricular activities. Perhaps I would not have been as outraged if the file was that of a woman who was already using the gateway drugs of alcohol and marijuana as a teenager, or of a girl who appeared to have no curfew and limited parental controls growing up. I would have expected the file to belong to one of the girls in my class who at fifteen and sixteen years of age flaunted the fact that they were dating men in their twenties and thirties. In essence, the sociologist in me wanted to confirm what I had learned about the predictors of negative outcomes for high-risk youth, and in this way, I remained stunned that the client file didn't belong to any of the girls having the high-risk behavioral patterns that are often discussed as the precursors to adult high-risk behavior. For a brief moment, I even realized that this could have been my file.

This file, however, belonged to Nicole, a classmate I met in the eighth grade when I sat next to her in the clarinet section for both marching band and concert band seasons. In fact, during band competition, Nicole played an alto clarinet solo that received high praise from the judges and our fellow bandmates. Nicole sang inspirational solos at many school assemblies, and I typically introduced the guest speaker. Right before the speaker would take to the podium, Nicole would render a motivational song—no easy feat in an inner-city school where the students were sitting on the edge of their seats to imitate the *Show Time at the Apollo* audience when they boo performers that fail to measure up. But Nicole had a beautiful soprano voice that only drew praise and applause at the end.

In addition to her strength as a soloist, Nicole grew up in a neighborhood church, and her mother worked as a paraprofessional at our school and was relatively active in the school's PTA. However, reflecting back, I do recall some hints of low self-esteem in Nicole's life. Nicole had a very bad skin problem and appeared to go overboard to be accepted by the "in-crowd." I remember as freshmen during band hazing week, she was the only freshman to follow through on the ridiculous requests and assignments given to us by the upperclassmen. Perhaps her unaddressed issues concerning self-esteem might explain why, after leaving our Rough-like community in pursuit of higher education, Nicole would succumb to peer pressure within the drugging and drinking community. In our inner-city school Nicole and I were among seven students in a graduating class of 145 that would at least start college in the fall of 1986. As I left for Texas Christian University in Fort Worth, Texas, Nicole remained local and attended a historical black college on the edge of the Rough, and unfortunately found herself in the heart of the Rough and fully participating in the high-risk behavior that she had managed to avoid for at least the first eighteen years of her life.

After getting over the initial shock and hurt of discovering Nicole's file, I finally got up the nerve to inquire about her whereabouts, as the outreach workers were known to maintain contact with the clients long after they left the HIP program. Although it was bittersweet news, I found some satisfaction in learning that Nicole had been in a drug rehabilitation program for the last twelve months. While I was relieved that Nicole was a success story in the HIP program, I was deeply disturbed and saddened that one of my classmates who had remained resilient in our Rough-like community had somehow ended up in the Rough. This feeling of despair prompted me to explore the theme of how girls from decent families find themselves facing the same Rough dilemmas that mainstream society continues to associate as negative, yet predictable outcomes primarily reserved for girls who grow up in the streets.

I felt relieved that the HIV prevention intervention had resulted in Nicole entering into a long-term drug treatment facility. Once I began transporting my own clients to drug treatment as part of the intervention process, one of the outreach workers arranged for me to see Nicole. She gave me a huge heartwarming hug and shared with me that the HIV prevention program had saved her life. Unfortunately, however, Nicole's file would not be the last one I would run across from my old classmates, as I would discover other clients who were high school cheerleaders, athletes, members of the academic top ten, and homecoming court queens. As I moved deeper into the Rough as an outreach worker and behavior interventionist, I discovered even more of my former schoolmates selling and using drugs, living in crack houses, and participating in sex work. For me, locating both categories of classmates sparked a sense of urgency that we must intervene in the lives of high-risk women at risk for HIV infection much earlier and more intensely.

Nicole's story resembles that of many of the women in this book who do not fit the stereotypical "bad girls to bad women" transition. Like Nicole, many of them grew up in relatively stable households where one or both parents worked. These women would not have been flagged as at-risk youth, as many of them participated in extracurricular activities, attended church, worked after school and in the summers, did not get pregnant in high school, received high school diplomas, and went on to be gainfully employed on living wage jobs.

At the same time, there is another group of women that was born into families that have been labeled at risk for two or more generations. Many are the offspring of prostitutes, pimps, drug dealers, and drug users, and having been born and raised in Rough-like environments, they grow up to view high-risk activities as the norm. In the end, however, no matter whether they grew up as decent or street girls, the women now find themselves living and coping to various degrees in this high-risk environment.

The challenge for HIV prevention researchers and practitioners is to face our collective reality that the faces and factors of new cases of HIV have changed, with current HIV prevention interventions programs underequipped to address the complexity of issues new clients present (Gilbert, 2003b). Rather than seek simple solutions, we must be willing to reach inside each woman and help her tell her own story in a way that empowers her to be a change agent in her own life. No longer can we afford to treat black women as a homogeneous group of high-risk women confined to high-risk communities. The challenge for the HIV prevention community is to invest in intervention processes that support examining each woman's unique background and circumstances that resulted in her present-day conditions. In an attempt to contribute to the theory and practice of such a paradigm shift in the HIV prevention community, I have included strategies and tactics at the end of each chapter in this book about how to respond to the unique differences that manifest among a group of women who have been objectified largely as a monolithic group of high-risk individuals.

BACKGROUND OF THE HEALTH INTERVENTION PROJECT

The ethnographic findings presented in this book are based on a larger study entitled The Health Intervention Project (HIP), which was implemented by Atlanta-based researchers with expertise in public health and sociological perspective. The HIP House—as it was affectionately known—addressed the idea that poor African-American women who smoke crack need more effective community-based (as opposed to institutionalized) HIV prevention programs to address their high-risk behaviors. Between 1997 and 2000, the staff enrolled over 400 drug-using African-American women from an at-risk neighborhood in Atlanta, Georgia, aiming to fill several gaps in HIV/AIDS prevention literature as it relates to the impact of race, class, and gender in the lives of poor African-American women who also use drugs and are at risk for HIV infection. An added benefit of having this program in the community was that it provided insight on how risk reduction programs both succeed and fall short in poor urban communities with scarce resources.

The women who participated in the ethnographic interviews were recruited from among a group of women who completed the HIP Project. The geographical location for the HIP House was initially an apartment in a housing project where the demographics of the residents matched those found in the census tract for this ghetto poor neighborhood. About two years into the study, the HIP House was relocated to a house approximately five blocks from the original apartment. At any given time, the core HIP House staff consisted of a program director, two to three interventionists, two interviewers, and two to three street outreach team members. Initially, evening and Saturday work were common. The schedule shifted as the project evolved and the staff changed. Toward the latter years, the HIP House operated Monday through Friday from 9:00 a.m. to 5:00 p.m. In addition to the full-time staff, there were several graduate students and community consultants who worked part-time over the course of the project. While there were key roles and responsibilities assigned to staff members, everyone participated in street outreach, as well as in food, clothing, and condom distribution (Sterk and Elifson, 2003).

The HIP risk reduction program was implemented in six key phases. The formative research, phase one, included a diverse team of street outreach workers, health educators, graduate students, and the co-primary investigators, who worked to develop a comprehensive perspective of members of the target population. In phase two, the street outreach team recruited high-risk African-American women to participate in the study. Next, phase three consisted of women participating in a baseline interview and pre- and posttest HIV counseling. They were then randomly assigned to one of three risk reduction interventions: a standard session or one of the two enhanced models known as the motivation, or negotiation, sessions. In phase four, women participated in a post intervention session administered after their intervention to determine short-term changes in high-risk behavior. Women were contacted six months after their intervention as part of phase five to measure longer term impacts of the HIV/AIDS prevention intervention. Phase six included the ethnographic interviews and a follow-up HIV test (Sterk and Elifson, 2003).

Each woman was given fifteen dollars for a baseline interview, twenty dollars after the post intervention interview, and twenty dollars for the six-month follow-up interview. The total monetary incentive for each woman completing the study was fifty-five dollars. No money was given for intervention sessions. However, the participants could request food, bus tokens, clothing, condoms, hygiene packets, or assistance with referrals during those appointments. In addition, program graduates were allowed one visit per month to get food and clothing. In the final phase of the project, forty-five women were asked to participate in a qualitative interview and were given an additional fifteen dollars. In addition, other incentives for women who allowed me to observe them in the field included cigarettes, condoms, food, and transportation to various social service providers.

ETHNOGRAPHIC RESEARCH METHODS

Participant Observation

Participant observation served as a key approach to observing and mapping risk in the Rough. This ethnography draws heavily on observations during my fieldwork as a graduate assistant and as an employee of the HIP Project. For the first four months I conducted baseline, post intervention, and six-month follow-up interviews. By my fifth month on the project, I became an interventionist responsible for my own clients. During my time at the study site, I helped distribute food, condoms, and clothing. In addition, I assisted some of the women in gaining access to various social services and community outreach programs. Over time, I became personally involved in some of the women's lives, including interactions with their extended families, steady partners, and children. In fact, I continue to maintain contact with some of the women I met during my time at the HIP House.

Participant observation also served as a key strategy for getting into the neighborhood after working hours. Extending my observations to weekends and evenings gave me more of an insider's perspective of the everyday realities of poor African-American women who use crack cocaine. Initially, I depended heavily on the street outreach team to introduce me to people in the area, and I adhered to whatever role they assigned me. Most of the time they presented me as a new "girl" at the HIP House who would be helping the women out.

Just as Whyte (1981) warned, it is far better to allow gatekeepers to introduce you and do the talking in the earlier periods of fieldwork. Once I had been associated with the HIP House for about three months, however, I was quite comfortable picking up clients and dropping them off alone, and I often used this time to establish rapport with the women. Most seemed disappointed to find out that I never used drugs and was not in recovery, but they continued to talk about past and present experiences. My lack of experience may have limited my ability to relate in some instances, but it also may have allowed some women to open up as they took it upon themselves to "school me" concerning the realities of street life. Even though most did so describing "other" women's behavior, such conversations provided an insider's perspective on general trends and patterns of everyday life in the Rough.

I was able to "code switch" depending on the field setting (Anderson, 1999). For example, among drug dealers who could help locate women, I took on the role of "concerned interventionist" willing to go into any crack house or rooming house to find a client for an appointment. As I was keenly aware of the perceived and real power the dealers have in the community and the danger they may pose for not respecting their "corner," I always made a point to talk to them and tell them exactly what I was doing.

In the evenings and on weekends I often played the role of "street-smart former housing-project girl," dropping names and mentioning associations with some of the "high rollers" with whom I grew up. Sometimes I just hung out on various corners with women from the HIP Project. Over time, the drug dealers were comfortable with me and proceeded to transact business in my presence. In any case, I was careful to downplay any connection with drug treatment or pass any moral judgment on the activities I observed, as this may have resulted in cold treatment or maltreatment if the dealers had taken my comments personally or felt I had the potential to hurt their business.

In my initial association with the HIP House, I had no intention of using my research experiences as the basis for a dissertation project. I had come to graduate school to study and improve the lives of at-risk youth. After looking on the GSU Web site, I came across the work of my dissertation chair, Dr. Kirk Elifson. I was drawn to his work because I was familiar with the geographical location. I had no formal training in HIV/AIDS research or drug abuse, nor did I have formal fieldwork training. I simply wanted to work on an applied research project. I e-mailed him explaining my desire to learn more about his project. He responded and suggested that I meet with him and the co-primary investigator, Dr. Claire Sterk, who also was one of my dissertation committee members. After that meeting, I visited the HIP House and met the project director and other staff members. The project director asked me why I wanted to work there. I responded naively, "because I want to help these women."

I say naively, because my agenda was to get as many of them to drug treatment as I could. I wanted to touch and change lives. I had no idea what the research project entailed and that my personal agenda—if carried out—would actually have been in conflict with the study design. But, that didn't stop me in the early months of the study. In fact, my personal goals resulted in the entire staff having to go through a day of retraining where the interventionists voiced their frustrations with my approach to "preaching" to the women about drug treatment prior to their intervention. The primary investigators agreed to allow me to continue working there and I agreed to not speak of treatment until after a woman had completed her six-month follow-up. However, as an interventionist, I could assist my own clients within the guidelines of the research project. This consisted mainly of waiting until the women initiated a discussion about drug treatment.

At this point I had no particular theoretical framework for my dissertation project. I was taking a class on grounded theory and had worked with secondary text to build theory. I now wanted to conduct a research project in which I used my own interviews to build theory. After discussing my goals and interests with the primary investigators, I was assigned the task of conducting qualitative interviews for understanding the women's perceptions of the risk reduction process. We agreed on an interview guide that would serve a dual purpose: (1) investigate the intervention process from the women's perspective and (2) serve as a first step in learning more about how these women cope with multiple oppressions.

In-Depth Interviews

The in-depth interview was used to understand how at-risk women make sense of their lives and behavior within the context of risk reduction and an at-risk environment. In addition, I was able to inquire about behaviors, people, and places I observed in the Rough. Each woman was given a brief overview of the qualitative interview process. I began by introducing myself, followed by informing women they had been selected to provide more details about their risk behavior and life in general. I gave some details about my background as a product of the inner city and tried to present myself as someone genuinely interested in helping women in the neighborhood. In some cases I talked about the fact that I had never personally done or been addicted to drugs, yet my family had been greatly impacted by the crack cocaine epidemic. In other situations, the women asked me questions about my life. Still other women interjected and started the interviews by recalling some interaction they had with me earlier. Those who had been my clients typically updated me on their areas of progress as well as setbacks. There were a few whose family and children I had met over the course of the intervention and I was sure to ask about them.

The interview guide served as a key tool for the in-depth interviews. I used it as a guide only, with the understanding that not every question was relevant to each woman. To be clear, I had memorized many of the questions from the interview guide by about the twenty-fifth (of forty-five) interview and was able to focus on the participant as opposed to "my questions." In fact, in the last eight interviews, I did not use the interview guide to collect data. I asked the women to talk about themselves and the interview flowed from wherever their conversations began (Gentry, Elifson, and Sterk, 2005).

I informed each woman that she would be compensated fifteen dollars for her time and could request to end the interview or make statements off the record at any time. Interviews lasted between forty-five minutes and two hours. The average length was approximately one hour. The process began with a verbal reiteration of the informed consent, as each woman had previously signed a consent form at the beginning of the study. While this form included the women's consent for every phase of the study, I discussed the key differences between this interview and the others to ensure that they knew they were being taped. All forty-five interviews were tape recorded and transcribed verbatim. The use of the tape recorder was discussed with each participant at the beginning of the interview. While they were encouraged to view the machine as an aide, they were given the option of refusing to be taped. Throughout most of the interviews, the respondents periodically glanced at the recorder, particularly when discussing participation in illegal and other high-risk activities. This may be due in part to the emphasis I placed on being willing to allow them to talk "off record" about sensitive issues. I was careful to balance giving enough information to make each woman feel comfortable talking to an outsider about her private life, while keeping questions brief enough to avoid prompting for a particular response. For example, I did not want the women to feel that I was searching for answers that they were drug free and in monogamous relationships (Gentry, Elifson, and Sterk, 2005).

Generally, after an hour clear patterns emerged concerning particular lifestyles. As suggested by Berg (2001), social life operates within fairly regular patterns that allow for the general classification of things, persons, and events. For the women in this study, those "emerging patterns" centered on the day-to-day life on and off the streets, sex work, intimate partners, housing arrangements, family backgrounds and upbringings, HIV risk factors, and drug use (Gentry, Elifson, and Sterk, 2005).

In some cases, I would like to have continued probing on areas of interest, but interviewing drug users can be challenging. Some participants were fatigued from their prior night's activity. One participant showed up immediately after having engaged in excessive substance use. After attempting to talk with her for a few minutes, we both agreed that she should be rescheduled. She returned the next day and completed a one-hour interview (Gentry, Elifson, and Sterk, 2005).

Some elected to speak off record, mainly about criminal activity, welfare issues, rape, and the ways in which they lost their children. I honored these requests every time. For that reason, five of the transcribed interviews were much shorter than the others, yet I have additional notes concerning the off-record conversations. This resulted in ten typed pages of notes—approximately two pages per off-the-record interview (Gentry, Elifson, and Sterk, 2005).

The interviews were conducted in the same setting as the intervention sessions. Upon arriving in the room for their interviews, several women commented on remembering their sessions having been in the same room. They immediately began to recall certain things that were important to them at the interview site. This assisted in establishing trust and rapport, as well as helping women recollect their experiences because they were familiar and comfortable with their surroundings (Gentry, Elifson, and Sterk, 2005).

HIV Testing Postintervention

The last thirty-three participants were asked to retake the HIV test. Two did not retest because they tested positive the first time. The first ten were not retested because it occurred to me after analyzing the first few interviews that these women were still displaying risky behavior to varying degrees and for a variety of reasons. Therefore, I asked the primary investigators to approve an HIV retest for the remaining qualitative interview participants. All of the retests were negative. I retested twenty-one of the thirty-three women, and an outreach worker assisted with the other twelve. For those I tested, I turned on the tape recorder during the HIV test to capture our conversations about the test and about AIDS in general. None of the thirty-three women was reluctant to take the test. Some began to open up during this process about the times they put themselves at risk; others were adamant about not having put themselves at risk and appeared almost proud to retest and "prove" to me that they were practicing safer sex. All of the women expressed a desire to know their results, and with the help of an outreach worker, I made an effort to recontact them. However, not all women were accessible, despite having provided clear directions on where to find them. I personally delivered eight test results; and other outreach workers assisted in delivering to seventeen women their test results. Eight women of the thirty-three did not receive their results.

THEORETICAL FRAMEWORK

Black Feminist Thought

I selected black feminist thought as a critical theory for interpreting the women's lives in a way that clarifies a standpoint for poor

African-American women in relation to the social, political, and economic issues that may impact their risk for HIV/AIDS (Collins, 2000). One of the key tenets of black feminism is its indictment of institutional practices. The unequal relationships that these practices represent are what Collins (2000) implies are legitimate issues for black feminist theory to analyze and ultimately act upon. Black feminist thought as critical theory works to question the legitimacy of those social institutions that exploit black women or any other oppressed groups in our society. Existing and past institutional practices that place poor black women at risk for HIV/AIDS in high-risk environments fit black feminist criteria for social problems that should be addressed theoretically and practically (Gentry, Elifson, and Sterk, 2005).

Collins (1998) defines critical social theory as encompassing bodies of knowledge and sets of institutional practices that actively grapple with the central questions facing groups of people differently placed in specific political, social, and historic contexts characterized by injustice. Accordingly, critical theory is generally used to critique the ways in which people are constrained to act and to identify themselves in terms of particular social institutions. In *Black Feminist Thought*, Collins (2000) outlines a discourse for interpreting the experiences of African-American women by integrating the key works of several leading black feminist authors. Her thematic approach can be applied to understanding poor African-American women's lives in relation to HIV/AIDS intervention.

The first theme is that of self-definition and self-valuation. Collins (2000) conceptualized self-definition as "the idea of challenging the political knowledge-validation process that has resulted in externally defined, stereotypical images of African-American women and black womanhood." The second theme centers on black feminist thought as a sociological perspective that interconnects race, class, and gender as being equally oppressive in our society. The third theme is that a black feminist perspective is necessary in understanding the unique experiences of African-American women. The strength of this theme is its insistence that even women who practice so-called deviant behavior have a voice in black feminism. The fourth theme centers on the controlling images constructed for poor African-American women. The image of the "crack whore" emerged as a class-specific, controlling image placed on poor African-American women who trade sex for crack and money. Finally, black feminist thought provides a framework for examining structure and agency as a platform for social change. A structural argument shows the historical legacy of interlocking oppressions, focusing primarily on how, within hierarchical power relations, the ideas produced by elite groups about community, difference, voice, and justice are the ruling ideas. This fifth theme reflects a point of synergy between the experiences of African-American women and others that are at risk for HIV infection primarily due to social inequality.

Symbolic Interactionism

Symbolic interactionism is a theoretical perspective for understanding the processes, interactions, meanings, and interpretations of various social phenomena (Blumer, 1969). Specifically, it is concerned with what common set of symbols and understandings have emerged to give meaning to people's interactions (Patton, 1990). In addition, it provides guiding principles of qualitative inquiry for scholars who want to research and interpret human group life and human behavior. In *Symbolic Interactionism: Perspective and Method,* Blumer (1969) acknowledges that several leading scholars contributed to the intellectual foundation of symbolic interactionism, including Mead (1934), Thomas (1972), James (1890), and Cooley (1902).

Blumer (1969) conceptualizes the nature of symbolic interactionism as centered on three premises, including meanings, social interactions, and interpretations. All of these concepts are relevant in the process of reducing risk among a specific group of people. First, he argued that human beings act toward things on the basis of the meanings things have for them. Second, Blumer (1969) offers that meanings are social products that are formed through interaction with other people. Third, Blumer posits that meanings and interactions among individuals undergo an interpretative process, in which each person deals in varying degrees with things encountered in everyday life. Blumer further offered that interpretation should not be regarded as a mere automatic application of established meanings. He perceived interpretation as a formative process in which meanings are used and revised as instruments for the guidance and formation of action.

Symbolic interactionism offers an explanation for how individuals interpret and select for themselves the "slices" of behavioral change they will attempt generally based on their daily reality. In this case, the process of "slicing" behavioral change strategies is influenced by one's self-perceived reality as a poor African-American woman who smokes crack.

At the root of symbolic interaction is a desire to understand aspects of human groups and the ways in which these women go about life's activities (Blumer, 1969). In this way, symbolic interaction shares common theoretical premises with black feminist thought. Implicit in symbolic interactionism is the notion that one wants to understand a group's culture, including customs, traditions, norms, values, and rules. In addition, scholars of symbolic interactionism want to understand the impact of social structure—that is, the relationships derived from how people act toward each other based on social position, status, role, authority, and prestige—on a particular group of humans (LaRossa and Reitzes, 1994; Maines, 1989; Stryker, 1980).

Social Constructionist Perspective

The social constructionist perspective provides a theoretical framework for examining the objective and subjective realities of everyday life. In examining the social construction of high-risk environments, where risky drug and sexual behavior is objectified as the norm, researchers are able to explain the social context within which the HIV risk reduction intervention takes place. Berger and Luckmann (1966), who clarified a sociology of knowledge in their book, *The Social Construction of Reality: A Treatise in the Sociology of Knowledge,* argued that "the basic premise of reality as socially constructed is that truth and knowledge are discovered, made known, reinforced, and changed by members of society. As social beings, we respond to our interpretations and definitions of situations, not the situations themselves, thereby shaping reality."

Thus, prevention intervention program implementers must attempt to make some sense of the realities that shape the lives of the target population in order to be effective in getting high-risk participants to change their behavior. Likewise, the targeted population is trying to interpret the key points of risk reduction for themselves and in doing so shape their own reality about their risky behavior and their prospects for change. So, as those who practice high-risk behavior discover their own risk factors, they either defend their reality or attempt to change their reality.

Berger and Luckmann's theory of the social construction of reality is divided into three key components, each having relevance for the social construction of high-risk environments and high-risk behaviors. First, they discuss the foundation of knowledge in everyday life. Next, they examine society as objective reality in terms of how reality becomes institutionalized and legitimized over time and in space. Finally, they posit that society as subjective reality centers on the internalization of reality in primary and secondary socialization.

An understanding of everyday life as internal and external reality provides theoretical overlap between symbolic interactionism and social constructionism. A perspective of one's "total reality" is applicable to the case of crack-using women, as it highlights that the meaning of crack cocaine is internal for those who use the substance, and yet there is an external, albeit stigmatized reality of crack usage among those who do not use this drug. Berger and Luckmann lay the foundation for the social construction of reality by theorizing about the reality of everyday life. They perceive the reality of everyday life as an ordered reality. The authors build on this in the following quotation:

> Its [the reality of everyday life] phenomena are prearranged in patterns that seem to be independent of my apprehension of them and that impose themselves upon the latter. The reality of everyday life appears already objectified, that is constituted by an order of objects that have been designated as objects before my appearance on the scene. The language used in everyday life continuously provides me with the necessary objectifications and posits the order within which these make sense and within which everyday life has meaning for me. I live in place that is geographically designated; I employ tools . . . I live with a web of human relationships . . . which are also ordered by means of vocabulary. In this manner language marks the co-ordinates of my life in society and fills that life with meaningful objects. (1996, p. 21)

What Berger and Luckmann offer is that everyday life is organized around various social interactions and the language used to transmit meanings. Social interaction in everyday life has a profound impact on the process of risk reduction. It is tied to the key component of everyday life as structured both spatially and temporally. Time of day and place of risk, as well as time of day and place of intervention, are important elements of how people in high-risk environments create reality and respond to behavioral change.

In addition, spatial structure is a key component to the social construction of high-risk environments. If these women smoke crack in their own homes, they may have different experiences with risky behavior than those women who are forced or choose to smoke and trade sex in crack houses. Likewise, those who smoke outside on the streets may avoid some risk factors such as getting stuck in an unsafe crack house.

High-risk environments where individuals smoke crack and trade sex have a language and knowledge that is associated with everyday life for members of this group. Berger and Luckmann refer to this as "the common stock of knowledge." In the case of high-risk environments, common stock of knowledge includes what people believe about HIV/AIDS, what people believe about the risk of drug use and sexual behavior in relationship to HIV/AIDS, and what people believe about their chances of getting HIV/AIDS.

Summary of Theoretical Perspectives

The three theoretical frameworks presented in this chapter explain key aspects of the relationship between poor African-American women who use crack and the social structure within which they experience everyday life. Each theoretical framework that offers microsociological analysis of a particular social phenomenon should also include a perspective on the macrosociological structures within which a person experiences everyday life.

In addition, each theory provides a perspective of self, which has implications for HIV intervention in the life of the socially constructed poor African-American crack user. All three theories presented focus on some aspect of these individuals as capable of developing a capacity for thinking, defining, and self-reflecting. Each theoretical framework acknowledges to varying degrees that individuals shape their environments through their actions and reactions. Moreover, these women can radically alter their definitions of self and situations, and in doing so they can change their high-risk behavior. The specific focus of self for each theoretical framework includes symbolic interactionism's ideas about self-development, social constructionism's emphasis on the construction of an internal and external self, and black feminism's highlighting of the importance of self-definition and self-valuation.

Together these three theoretical frameworks offer a comprehensive perspective of how poor African-American women who use crack cocaine interact with others in high-risk environments. To be clear, each theoretical perspective has a different slant on the degree to which the interactions are actively constructed. Black feminist thought stands apart from the other theories because of its more radical discourse and synergy with other conflict perspectives. However, black feminism's core themes of self-definition and self-valuation provide a natural alliance with the other two theories.

In addition, these theories provide a framework for analyzing high-risk environments as social structures with a particular social order. Again, black feminism tends to focus more than the other theories on the powerful social forces as "shapers and maintainers" of the high-risk environments. As such, black feminism supports a school of thought that poor African-American women unconsciously relinquish their internal power to these external forces. Only by defining and placing a value on the self are African-American women able to reject objectified roles and replace them with more authentic ones.

While the other two theories focus on change through redefining situations, their general inclination to do so void of race, class, and gender sets them apart from black feminist thought. Also, black feminist thought views social institutions as more structurally situated than do the other theories presented in this chapter. Black feminism advocates that these social organizations do not change as a part of the natural order of society, but rather they must be changed via external pressure from those experiencing social inequality as a part of everyday life. In any case, all three perspectives have direct implications for attempting to change high-risk behavior in high-risk environments.

Each theory supports an ethnographic inquiry for exploring processes and meanings among individuals and social forces that help shape their lives. Symbolic interactionism focuses on interpreting the meanings, interactions, and processes associated with HIV prevention programs. The social constructionist perspective highlights how high-risk environments have an objective and subjective reality, along with the people and behaviors that are associated with such environments. Finally, black feminist thought clarifies key components of the first two theoretical frameworks from the standpoint of African-American women.

RESEARCH OBJECTIVES

The overall objective of this study was to gain an understanding of how poor African-American women who smoke crack cocaine reduce their risk for HIV infection. Several research questions guided the inquiry for accomplishing this objective: (1) What conditions and behaviors led to these women being labeled at risk for HIV/AIDS? (2) How do they interact in their present environment? (3) What strategies do they use to cope with being at risk for HIV/AIDS? and (4) What are the consequences of their participation in an HIV/AIDS prevention intervention?

The first question seeks to explore how these women came to be at risk for HIV/AIDS. Their perception of why and how they are at risk provides valuable information to HIV/AIDS prevention planners. The second question focuses on understanding their everyday lives as high-risk women living in a high-risk environment among other high-risk actors. The third question suggests that women are coping with their present situation, albeit on the margin, and that these coping skills can be enhanced to help women reduce their high-risk behavior. The fourth question implies that these women have agency and perceive themselves to be empowered to make changes in their behavior that may result in decreasing their risk for HIV infection. Together these questions are key in constructing implications for HIV prevention programs for poor African-American women who smoke crack.

Given the continued increase in the number of new cases of poor African-American women who use crack cocaine, we know that a simple transfer of risk reduction strategies is not the most effective method for reversing the trend among this high-risk group. For the most part, public health scholars and practitioners have ignored

African-American women's unique history when designing and implementing risk reduction. A careful examination and appreciation for African-American women's socialization in the United States would provide historical evidence as to how they survive and strategize despite pressure from oppressive forces (Gray-White, 1999; White, 1994). In essence, authentic voices of black women's risk and resilience are very much needed in HIV prevention.

Chapter 2

Living in the Rough

Every morning I get up and look in the mirror and I look at myself and I say, "hey, I like you." This is what I do every day. I take
my heart out my chest and put it in the dresser drawer. And once
you step out that door, anything goes in this neighborhood.

Dee-Dee, a 50-year-old crack cocaine user

Living arrangements emerged as a major theme early in my fieldwork, when, as an outreach team member, I had to become familiar
with the streets, houses, and hangout places throughout the neighborhood. For example, when picking women up for appointments and
dropping them off, I heard many of them comment about their living
arrangements, including who they lived with, others who were in the
house, or how long they had been there. Women who did not have
permanent addresses often provided the street names of the main cor-
ridors where we could usually find them for their appointments. I also
noticed that the women who lived in houses and apartments generally
wanted to return to the destination where we picked them up after
their intervention, whereas women we located in the streets were prone
to ask for rides to places other than their original location. I suspect
that over time the various social networks knew the purpose of the
HIP House and that we provided monetary stipends to participants.
Some women may not have wanted to return to the areas where there
was a high concentration of other street women as a way to avoid sharing their money or paying outstanding debts. These women's requests
for alternative drop-off places included other corners, the bus stop or

Black Women's Risk for HIV: Rough Living
© 2007 by The Haworth Press, Taylor & Francis Group. All rights reserved.
doi:10.1300/5784_02

25

transit system, or a relative's house, usually their mother. As the outreach team intensified its efforts to maintain contact with the women,
staff members asked direct questions such as "What streets do you
hang out on?" or "Which one of these corners do you hold up?" I recall one woman saying, "This my street right here; anytime you want
me, just come right here."

On the other hand, when we asked women with permanent addresses
where they wanted to be dropped off, many typically responded "take
me home" or "I am a house woman" or "the streets don't call me like
they do them [the street women]." Over the course of my fieldwork
I observed that several of the women—usually the "street women"—
changed living arrangements several times. I remember feeling frustrated that they were so difficult to locate, while the women in houses
seemed more stable. I started to question whether or not the women
in the streets were more at risk for HIV/AIDS in comparison with
those who had housing (Battle et al., 1995).

The typology of "street" and "house" women is used to describe the
patterns that were emerging during my fieldwork. These broad categories of street and house are further divided into subtypes that more
accurately described the diverse living arrangements among women
in the study. At least three of the women who are rooming housed are
also in steady-partner relationships; and three of the women who are
market renters have steady partners. At the same time, the steady-
partner housed may live in a rooming house or market rent house.
The difference is that women classified as rooming housed or market
renters who have live-in steady partners claim these men live with
them and cannot put them out. The steady-partner housed women, in
contrast, are primarily dependent on the income of their partners for
continued living arrangements.

STREET WOMEN

Street women fit the controlling images that society has socially
constructed for women addicted to crack cocaine. Their high-risk behavior is more public, as they can be observed in broad daylight solic-
iting sex or smoking crack on the streets in the Rough. They dress and
act in ways that uphold the social construction of the "crackhead" or
"crack whore." They may go days without personal grooming and

hygiene maintenance; paradoxically, they are still able to turn tricks even in this extreme physical state. As outreach workers and interventionists, there were many times we had to make the tough decision to "just leave them out there" because they were not willing or able to come in for appointments. The street women typically are the most socially isolated. They are detached from mainstream society in that they are jobless and homeless. They have little if any contact with their families, some by choice, and others by force. Street women typically have had their children taken away by social service authorities; however, many of the children remain with other family members.

Street women are highly likely to engage in street violence both as victims and initiators, particularly when money and drugs are involved. Thus, in comparison to house women, street women are likely to go to jail for fighting and prostitution much more frequently. In addition, street women had more encounters with rape at the hands of johns either getting physically violent or reneging on the agreement to pay for sexual services. Still other street women described escaping rape as a normal part of living in the Rough. The average street woman has been using crack cocaine between ten and fifteen years and has concluded that both outpatient and inpatient drug treatment programs simply have not worked for her in the past. To be clear, house women and street women alike engage in risky sexual behavior; however, street women discussed higher rates of unprotected vaginal sex with multiple partners than did house women.

As I began interacting more with women outside the HIP House, I discovered the complexities associated with subtyping. Not only did the women describe instances when they may have been one or more of the subtypes at any given time, it was clear that street women moved in and out of housing situations relatively frequently in comparison to house women. I have developed definitions and characteristics for three subtypes of street women that I believe represent a large part of what I observed over the two years I spent in the field: (1) the absolute homeless, (2) the hustling homeless, and (3) the rooming housed. While women in these subgroups have different experiences in the Rough, most share the reality of having to renegotiate their housing situations anywhere from several times a week to several times a month. In the case of the absolute homeless, they may find themselves negotiating sleeping arrangements on a daily basis.

Even the rooming housed women, who have the most stability of all street women, acknowledge that their average length of stay in one house is three to four months. Their constant change is generally due to lacking money when rent is due. Therefore, they are evicted fairly frequently, as they have little negotiating power with rooming house managers and owners who seldom tolerate people remaining in the room beyond a week if they fail to pay their rent. Some rooming housed women confided that they often smoke up their already meager income, believing they can make up the difference by hustling. Others who work point to having been between jobs or sick and under the doctor's care when they were evicted for nonpayment. Only one woman had been a tenant in the same rooming house for more than a year.

While women have a variety of experiences in the Rough, one's perception of reality often drives risk behavior. For example, Tracie, a 37-year-old sex worker, believes that she must take a chance with any man that comes along. As a street woman who also performs sex work, she perceives herself to be at the mercy of paying customers. She stresses, "I catch whatever comes along . . . whoever looking for a date. Do whatever it is he needs me to do, get the money and go and just pray this brother don't have AIDS."

Tracie described what it is like every day in the Rough as a street woman and how such living arrangements translate into risk. Like Tracie, other street women are exposed to multiple sex partners with varying requests for sex acts that may or may not include condom use. In addition, depending on how desperate they are, women like Tracie may have to perform more sex acts to make sufficient money if they are negotiating with customers who sense they will perform for a lower amount of money.

The Absolute Homeless

Perhaps the most desperate of the three types of street women were those I classified as absolute homeless. The women grouped as absolute homeless literally live on the streets, and describe themselves as having no place to go. They leave their possessions wherever they can and often lose what little personal property they are able to maintain on the streets. Sometimes they take refuge in shelters, but for various reasons are highly likely to take their chances on the streets. This group is least likely to have biological relatives living in the Atlanta area, and therefore they rely on others in the drug scene to provide social, economic, and emotional support. The absolute homeless pay for almost everything in the high-risk environment. They pay people who own houses to wash their clothes, provide a meal, or for a place to sleep for anywhere from a few hours to one night. The women who have houses in the Rough generally are the ones who provide these services to the absolute homeless, and have been known to put a price tag on everything from a quarter for a cigarette to fifty cents to use the restroom indoors. I wrote in my field notes:

> I can't believe how they pimp each other. Dee-Dee [a steady-partnered, housed] charges the girls for every little thing she does for them. She says they steal it right back. I guess I can see her point though—why give them free meals, wash their clothes, and stuff when they just smoke up their money in dope. In some ways she is trying to make them responsible for their own care. I wonder if Dee-Dee gives out the condoms from the HIP House like she said . . . who I am kidding . . . I know she sells them . . . and to the people who need them the most, which are the girls on the street.

At least four women in this study talked about their lives as absolute homeless women. Portia, a 34-year-old crack smoker, had physical and facial features that challenged the stereotypical image of street women as "crackheads." When I met her she was living with a steady partner who sold and used drugs. About three months after I met her, the apartments they lived in were condemned and everyone was ordered to move out by the end of the month. Her steady partner's family took him in, but due to a history of violence and abuse between the two, the family would not allow Portia to live with them. Her mother is a social worker living in "Mexico State," and having no family in Atlanta, she took to the streets. When I saw her on the streets I almost didn't recognize her because she was not as neat and tidy as when she lived in an apartment, and had begun to show some physical attributes often reserved for the "crackhead." I stopped the car and asked her if she wanted to do an interview. She said she could come right then and jumped in the car. I asked her about life now that she was out of the violent relationship. She replied, "I really have nothing. I live in nothing. I don't have no apartment. I be here and there. I just have good friends who let me kick it and keep my clothes."

Having no family of her own in the area resulted in Portia becoming absolutely homeless. She began living on the streets and performing high-risk sex in order to survive. I asked her if she could go home, and she tearfully stated that she had run every con game imaginable on her mother and didn't believe living with her would be an option. Now Portia has been homeless for six months and has intensified her role as a sex worker, replacing her previous one of selling drugs with her former steady partner. This change of work has resulted in higher risks for HIV, as Portia no longer has a steady supply of drugs and stable living arrangements.

Mona, a 40-year-old crack user, describes what it is like to be absolutely homeless for a longer period of time. Unlike Portia, who has been homeless for less than a year, Mona spent almost ten years as an absolute homeless woman. She described herself as a mentally ill person who will not take her medicine or cooperate with the mental health agency for fear of being institutionalized. Instead, she opted to live under a bridge with others also seeking to avoid the authorities. She recalls life prior to her association with the HIP House:

> Let me see. I was homeless then. I'd get up and go to the Day Shelter and take me a shower and get me something to eat. I was working at McDonald's then. I would come back and get my uniform. I think I was working evenings then. I was the only woman down there (under the bridge) for a long time. I collected cans. I wasn't too much into doing stuff illegal. The only thing I was doing illegal was the drugs. Then at night we'd get together and get some lumber. Some of us had jobs where they collect wood. Everybody was pretty much together doing something so we all could survive.

Mona went on to say that there were about twenty-five men and women living under this bridge for almost a decade. Mona described how individuals who are homeless try to maintain relationships. Relationships that house women tend to take for granted place absolute homeless women at higher risk for HIV, as condom use is not a priority in this state of everyday living. Mona herself admitted that she failed to maintain condoms and thus rarely used them with paying and steady partners whom she met under the bridge. In addition, Mona discussed how many people under the bridge inject drugs. Mona was not part of this subgroup and could not comment on whether or not they shared needles.

However, if condoms were scarce in this environment, I would presume that those needing clean needles would face similar dilemmas. To complicate the level of risk, homeless IDUs (injection drug users) also interact with noninjection drug users. If they had sexual relations with IDUs, then noninjection drug users became even more vulnerable for the spread of HIV/AIDS. Thus, while Mona did not associate with this group during the times that they may have been injecting drugs, if she later had unprotected sex with someone from this group, then her risk factors increased.

I asked her if they used condoms during that time and she responded that they did when a community outreach program (other than HIP) would come and pass them out and check them for HIV. I assume it was a program with a research component because Mona described it as one that "paid them to participate." But as Mona reflected on those under the bridge she believed to be HIV positive and in her estimation "possibly having full-blown AIDS," these condom outreach efforts may have been too little too late. According to Mona, "I think about the people that I had seen that had gotten AIDS over the years and had died. They face, everything, start changing and the first thing they do is get white around the mouth . . . skin start peelin' around their mouth and around they nose and they started lookin' old and eyes start sinking back in their heads."

Like Mona, many street women attempt to identify HIV-positive men by physical signs that they may be infected. It was common to find both street and house women describing what they perceived to be the physical symptoms of HIV/AIDS in others. However, by the time physical signs manifest, the person could have had the virus for a long period of time and have infected numerous partners, especially those who take risk based on a person's physical appearance.

While Mona described her homeless experience as one with little or no violence, other homeless women provided less than positive accounts of their time on the streets. In fact, with the exception of

Mona, all the other absolute homeless women had been raped, severely beaten, or narrowly escaped an attacker on the streets.

Dorothy, a 41-year-old recovering crack user, described being a homeless sex worker in the Rough. She had one month in recovery when I met her, but recalled that the entire time she was associated with the HIP House she was homeless. As a homeless sex worker she tried to practice safe sex, but admitted that it was very hard to be consistent.

> Really I wasn't fixin' to put nobody thang in my mouth without no condom, but I can't say that I didn't do it. I did, but I tried so very hard to practice. I put myself in some situations. One time I was in a dangerous situation where I feared for my life. I went and got the weed for them and when I got back in the car one of the boys pulled a knife to my throat and the thing of it was they didn't want anything from me. They didn't want no sex. It was just a thrill. But it was one li'l guy that was sitting in the back seat he say, "Don't do that shit man." He say, "Stop that bull shit." He talking about, "Naw, I want her to give me some head." Then I say, "Well okay, I'll do that. Just please take that knife from my . . ." I say, "Please please just don't hurt me."

As a homeless sex worker, Dorothy went about her daily routine of turning tricks and doing drugs. She discussed finding herself in an abandoned house that, in the early stages of her drug use, she vowed never to end up in. She elaborated on the fact that she even made a cardboard box her home in an attempt to avoid the "stink house." However, Dorothy reflects on how she placed herself at risk for HIV infection during the time she was homeless. According to her, several members of her social network recently died from AIDS.

> There was an empty house and it was so stink. I used to pass that house and I said I would never go in there. The Red Dogs [Atlanta's special drug police unit] came in there and busted it one time and said, "I ain't even gone take ya'll ass to jail." He said he wouldn't even gonna take us to jail. They wouldn't even come in. They said, "If ya'll wanna stay up in that shit, stay in there." And he talked about us so bad. He said, "Ya'll don't know who been in there with AIDS. Ya'll in there and shit all on

the floor." And it was. It was stink and it was all kind of germs going around there. And we didn't care; we were breathing that stuff in. I didn't care. I had to have some more dope. I was sleeping outside in a cardboard box. I had made me a little hut in a cardboard box. And people around me were dying fast. Three of my friends died last summer, and that's scary. I was afraid because we was in that cycle and we was in a circle. I was just so afraid that I had been with some of them folks that they had been with. And chances are that I had been, but since then I've had two negative HIV test.

Like Dorothy, other absolute homeless women frequently take chances that put them at risk for HIV infection. The key factors that distinguish absolute homeless women from others include (1) being on the streets for longer periods of time, (2) lacking family support in the area, and (3) frequently ending up in more isolated areas. While women in other groups may also face these dilemmas at some stage in their lives, the absolute homeless describe themselves as grappling with these issues on a daily basis, with very few exceptions.

The Hustling Homeless

The hustling homeless were another distinct group of street women. The one factor that distinguishes the hustling homeless from the absolute homeless is that the hustling homeless claim to be on the street even though they can go home to their families and become family housed. Unlike the absolute homeless who lack family support, the hustling homeless assert that their families will allow them to come home at any time if they would stop using drugs. There were five street women who described themselves as homeless "because they want to be out there." Most defended their families much in the same way as Yolanda does:

I got my whole family mad at me. They don't like it, you know but I can go home. My mama say you can bring your stuff home but there ain't nothin' out there in Decatur you know. I got to be me. My money ain't there. They just hate I'm on it [drugs] 'cause they feel that's what got me out here. That's what got me not wanting to come home and stuff, you know—like I ain't got no family. My mama say, it ain't like you ain't got no family that don't love you.

The hustling homeless frequent a type of house that is generally associated with a constant flow of traffic connected to drug using, drug selling, and sex work. These houses are often referred to as "whore houses" or "crack houses." The hustling homeless are described by others in the Rough as "out there," meaning they are perceived as doing drugs and performing sex all day and all night. Some even refer to them as "24/7" implying that they are drugging twenty-four hours per day and seven days per week. When they do take a break, it is only for a couple of hours or perhaps a few days. During this time they may become "daily" room renters paying anywhere from three to five dollars for a couple of hours or seven to ten dollars per night for a room on average. According to several accounts, the hustling homeless may have "thousands of dollars" in the morning because of a good drug hustle the night before. However, by the next night they could be penniless, and thus unable to pay for a room.

I generally found these hustling homeless women in rooming houses that are reserved for women who work as sex workers. House managers confirmed that some women live in their houses, while others rent rooms by the hour or by the day. The rooming house managers who allow women to live there admit the women must be willing to perform sex work, serving whatever clientele comes to the house.

In addition, several cars tend to frequent these types of rooming houses at the lunchtime and evening hours. I observed license plates from various suburban counties throughout the metropolitan area. The men often have wedding bands and drive luxury automobiles, substantiating these women's claims that their clientele consists mainly of middle-class married men from other neighborhoods. Some men come in work uniforms and others come in suits, particularly during the lunch hour. It is difficult to tell whether they are buying sex or drugs, or both. The men who enter the rooming houses first approach the house manager, who also may be dealing drugs. If they are regulars, they may request a woman they know in the house. New customers quickly ask the house manager for a woman willing to do certain sexual acts or may request a woman who has particular physical features. For example, they may ask for a "redbone," which is a lighter skinned African-American woman. Others prefer "big tits" or "big legs." In any case, the manager's role is to seek out girls with the requested physical attributes, as well as those willing to perform the requested sexual acts. Money is exchanged before the customer proceeds to the room. If he wants to get high or to drink, he is responsible for supplying these items.

Like the absolute homeless, the hustling homeless are more prone to street violence and attacks by men they describe as strangers to the Rough. As "seasoned" hustlers, these women generally perceive themselves to be in a position to handle such encounters. However, Janice, a 30-year-old crack user, describes how she fought to avoid rape. Her story is typical of others I heard from hustling homeless women.

> Well we had a li'l living room outdoors. I was out there by myself. I was feeling good and high. [I] took the last little hit. [I] seen this guy just kept walking around. I had never seen him before. He say, me and my uncle fixing on the house down the street. We getting high, you know ain't nobody but me and my uncle. I went on behind him (followed behind him). We gets in (the house) he reached like he fixin' to pay me, pull out a knife, put it around my neck, (and tells me to) get in the hole. I was like, please use a rubber. He slipped and laid the knife down and took off his clothes. I grab the knife. I wouldn't let that go for nothing in the world. I was bleeding everywhere from scrapes and stuff. We went on for about thirty or forty minutes where he trying to get that knife from me. Thank God, that would have been the only time I got raped. I went back up there where I started, where I met him at, where all the. . . . I ain't gone say friends, but smoke buddies and stuff at. And told them what happened and stuff right. All of them were saying call the police. Really I was on my own. Everybody be like, what you should have did. They saying the bad part. . . . You know, like you shouldn't have went with him. You shouldn't have did this or you should have. . . . Just all on my case. I'm all fucked up you know.

Janice's story highlights the similarities between the narratives of the women who were either raped or escaped rape, in that they generally were high on crack cocaine and at a point where they were desperate for another hit. As Janice described, having very few options for getting more drugs, she took a chance on leaving a familiar territory to follow a stranger to an abandoned house. Even after recognizing that she didn't know him, she took a chance that he may have just wanted a woman to get high with.

Another key point that Janice mentioned is she begged her attacker to use a condom. Many women who are raped report their attacker did not use a condom. A rapist's decision not to use a condom could be an indicator that he may be infected with HIV and has nothing to lose by not using a condom. Particularly, a rapist's decision to choose victims from among women who are sex workers and living on the streets but not use a condom himself suggests that he may already be HIV-infected. On the other hand, his decision could reflect the perception among some men in the neighborhood that women cannot give a man HIV. This group of misinformed men believes that only a man can "shoot" HIV into a woman.

Since Janice's partner has been in jail and is now in drug treatment, Janice has intensified her "hustle with dope boys" as a way of survival and to avoid sex work if she can. In her estimation, it is less risky to sell dope than have sex. Janice turns about ten "dates" per day and estimates that only five of them use a condom. I asked her why the other five do not use them. She said either they don't want to use them or didn't have any. She explains, "I suggest a rubber at all times, but by me just wanting the money and stuff—temptation—the dope, I just take a chance. But I'm strictly safe . . . try to be safe . . . boy I try."

Janice's dilemma in negotiating condom use mirrors that of women in general. Women can suggest condom use; however, men historically yield more power under such circumstances. Janice's power to walk away from noncomplying partners is weakened by her admittance that she needs the money. Judging from her comments, she is torn between trying to be safe and taking a chance to get money for drugs. Her intent to be safe is encouraging and serves as a starting point for an interventionist to help Janice move from the intention to be safe to the act of being safe. Janice described how she attempted to avoid unsafe sex prior to intervention. Her strategy of working with the drug dealers to make money helped her avoid having to turn dates. However, she admits that she takes risks in having unprotected sex if offered the right financial rewards. In further probing, I learned that her risk taking is mainly related to times when she is desperate and thus even a low amount of money becomes "the right financial reward."

Janice realizes that she is disadvantaged in hustling her knowledge because she uses drugs. Therefore her preferred hustle of selling drugs and overcharging naive customers sometimes leaves her having to resort to high-risk sexual behavior. She recalls how sometimes she would have "lots of money" and then in the next few hours find herself literally performing sex without condoms for two dollars. I asked her how often she finds herself in this predicament.

> Plenty of time it be worth it. Plenty of times for nothing. But I deal with it though. I don't look down. I keep my head up all the time. I don't let it get me down 'cause I had a choice, I had a choice to say no. Nobody didn't make me do it. Nobody didn't put a gun to my head or all that, I had a choice, so I learn to keep my head up.

Janice constantly finds herself coping with the idea that putting herself at risk may or may not yield the financial benefits she is seeking. Yet, even as a poor African-American woman who smokes crack, she finds enough esteem to keep her head up. This source of self-strength appears to stem from her belief that she is empowered to say no. Despite her daily life as a high-risk woman navigating a high-risk environment, Janice is adamant that she is to blame for her predicament. While this is a much-needed mind-set to facilitate change behavior, it also represents a lack of consciousness on her part about the social conditions that may hinder her ability to change. Like Janice, when other women who face intersecting race, class, and gender inequalities fail at changing behavior, they often blame themselves, when in fact several oppressive forces limit their abilities to make changes in their high-risk behavior.

I learned firsthand how the hustling homeless live their everyday life as I became acquainted with Valerie, a 32-year-old mother of six. Valerie is now a sex worker and in her own terms, "one of the baddest out there." I remember the day she first came to the HIP House. She was dirty, hungry, and loud. I was drawn to her because she was funny and not offensive in her outspoken demeanor. After her first session, she was given a stipend, and she asked me to take her to her mother's

house so she could give the money to her 14-year-old daughter to purchase a perm for her hair. When we arrived, we learned that her daughter had gone to spend the night with a relative in a housing project
about five miles away. Valerie demanded that someone call her daughter on the phone. In some ways, I felt that her outrage may have been
to convince me that she had some level of parental controls and could
locate her children instantly.

Once the daughter was on the phone, Valerie began shouting and
cursing her out saying, "Didn't Mama tell you to bring your ass home
and watch these children yesterday. . . . I'm gonna whip your ass when
I see you. . . . If my counselor bring me over there I am coming to get
you now." During the time Valerie is on the phone, her older brother is
inquiring intensely about who I am. He thought I was a social worker.
I wrote, "I really tried to ignore 'Eddie' as it was obvious why Valerie
chooses to stay in the streets." He is mean and nasty toward her.
I hated to hear him tell her she ain't going to never be shit. He pointed
to the family cat, which had two kittens, and asserted, "She (the cat)
take care of hers better than she [Valerie] do." I was proud of Valerie
for ignoring him. He made a point to tell me that he takes care of
Valerie's children while she runs the streets. He further clarified that
he drinks and smokes, but he takes care of his responsibilities. He
asked me if I was married and when I answered no, he asked me to go
to dinner with him. I politely declined.

In the meantime, Valerie came to ask me to go get her daughter and
bring her home. I smiled and said that I would under one condition
and that was that she reconsider her promise to whip her. I even offered that maybe she didn't come home because she didn't have bus
fare or a ride. Valerie agreed and we picked her daughter up. "Kenya"
was so cute and nice. Kenya and I developed a bond that resulted in
her coming to my house, going to a family wedding with me, and grad-
ing my papers over the summer.

I was also taking a graduate course called "Girls" where we were
taking a more intense look into the lives of high risk girls across race,
class, and gender lines. As part of the class I mentored Kenya and she
participated in my class assignment. During the interview, Kenya
commented about her mother's lifestyle and helped shape a perspective of the "hustling homeless" for me. She confirmed my earlier
thoughts that Valerie remains on the streets to avoid conflict with her

brother, who also smokes crack. Kenya often gets into trouble with her grandmother because she sneaks food out of the house and rides her bike to carry it to her mother. Kenya talked about being embarrassed walking home from school with friends and trying to avoid seeing her mother in the streets. She described making detours to avoid such encounters. In fact, she has gotten into fights at school defending her mother when other children make fun of her. Valerie's mother allows her to come home when she wants to; however, according to Kenya, this may happen for a night or so approximately once per month.

Over the next two months I learned much about how Valerie became a hustling homeless woman in the Rough, as she became one of my evening and weekend gatekeepers for observing the Rough beyond a Monday through Friday, nine-to-five routine. Valerie was raised by both of her parents, whom she described as hardworking people. She was never really interested in school and when a "slick talking" young man from the neighborhood approached her in the mid-1980s, she took to the streets to keep up with him. She jokingly recalls how she thought he would become a kingpin in the crack cocaine market. After she had her first child by him, she was no longer his "leading lady," and at eighteen years of age had to go on public assistance and move into a nearby public housing project.

"Leading lady" is synonymous with "main girl," and refers to a woman who is generally perceived to be the steady partner of the drug dealer. He may have other women whom he has sex with or who sell drugs for him, but the "leading lady" is generally the one who provides the foundation of a traditional home life for the drug dealer. She cooks, cleans, cares for children, and holds money for the drug dealer. Some leading ladies may hold drugs but rarely do they sell them as well. According to drug dealers, this woman is similar to the stay at home mother/wife image often depicted in Mafia movies.

As Valerie acknowledged, however, she resented and resisted the idea of being a stay-at-home woman. She liked the streets and wanted to be with her partner. After the first relationship failed, she tried to work a "decent" job at a nearby college as a custodian. However, she had grown accustomed to the fast money and perceived fun in the streets. In addition, she began selling drugs on the side to make ends meet. Valerie explained that the money came easy and before she knew it she was hanging with the high rollers, this time not as a girlfriend, but as a colleague and competitor. During that time she met another drug dealer who promised her the same type of lifestyle as her first drug-dealing partner had. Her first daughter had gone to live with her paternal grandparents, and for the most part Valerie was single and attractive. At this time she claims she was only a social drinker and had not begun to use drugs. She had another daughter (Kenya) with this man, and like the first one, the relationship went bad once the child was born. She said that depression set in and she began smoking drugs and hanging out all night. During this time she gave birth to two more children.

Valerie confided that there were nights she left Kenya at eight years of age in the house with her two smaller children. Before the authorities were notified, however, the local housing authority announced that it would be tearing down the housing projects. She was given $600 to move within a month. Now, with three children and a small stipend, she went back to her parents' home to what she described as a crowded household. "I started hanging in the street 'cause it was just too many grown folks in mom's house."

She took to the streets each night in search of "peace and quiet." According to Valerie, over time the streets and the street life became more of a place of freedom from the chaos of the home. However, Valerie readily admitted that there is something different about the streets today than ten years ago when she first began "ripping and running."

> It's just a lot of shit done changed. This shit ain't like it used to be where you can just get your shit and go about your business. Shit, now you got [men] selling [men]. Somebody putting their mister good bar into some peanut butter.

As Johnsie similarly acknowledges, "I had a place to stay, but then again I didn't. I had to pay somebody if I wasn't at my mom's house to stay at their house and it was hard if I didn't have the money." In some ways, women in this group challenge Liebow's (1993) analysis of homeless people as disadvantaged people overwhelmingly from poor families. Four of the five hustling homeless are from solidly middle-class African-American families. Johnsie's mom is a registered nurse and has a home in a predominantly white suburb where she cares for several of her grandchildren. Johnsie says she can go home at any time if she stops doing drugs. In the meantime, she places herself at risk for HIV by having to negotiate her sleeping arrangements daily. Like Johnsie, other women in this group confirm that they are from strong decent families who will allow them to come home any time they are ready to give up smoking crack.

Johnsie, who classified herself as high risk, based on not using condoms during oral sex, provides a perspective that represents women who attempt to avoid sex altogether, but still get the money or drugs. Johnsie rationalizes, "I know that's dirty, but if I can see where I don't have to lay down or give them some head or something like that and he just like crack much as I do, boy it's on."

Teresa's family owns several businesses in the inner city, including a day care center. Teresa's parents still live in the Rough as homeowners. Both Teresa and Johnsie sometimes venture home when they have money to give to their mothers in support of their children. But, for the most part, the hustling homeless remain on the streets and away from their families for extended periods of time.

The hustling homeless are generally cited as the hardest to reach subgroup in HIV prevention intervention. They appear to believe that they are extremely lucky and skillful as street women. While they like the attention and "freebies" associated with the HIP House, their stories were the most inconsistent in comparison to other groups. Yet, they are unique from other street women in that their families refuse to give up on them. Despite the games, lack of mothering to their minor children, and continued life as the fastest of all, the mothers of these women in particular continue to have hope that they will change.

The Rooming Housed

The final group of street women is the rooming housed. It may appear at first to be a paradox that a group of street women are housed. However, as I discovered over the course of my fieldwork, on any given day, members in this group can be homeless and back on the street. The rooming housed are not literally homeless; however, their housing situation must be negotiated on a monthly, weekly, and in some instances, daily basis. If they cannot maintain the rent, they are quickly evicted. This ability to pay is tied to their ability to earn money on a consistent basis. As many of them do not earn enough to escape poverty, they place themselves at risk in an effort to meet their daily needs.

Rooming houses can range from two to five bedrooms. Most occupants are adult men and women. Several women, however, have children and grandchildren who visit them in their rooming houses, but there were none in this study attempting to raise children on a daily basis in the rooming house environment. Rent for rooms depends on the quality of the room and other amenities associated with the room. For example, rooms with central heating and air generally are considered high-quality rooms and one can expect to pay seventy-five to eighty-five dollars per week depending on other factors, including room security and furnishings. Most have only one common kitchen area and one bathroom per house. Some rooming houses have central heating and air, while others leave it to the individual room renters to supply themselves with fans in the summer and space heaters in the winter.

The eleven women in this study who are classified as rooming housed highlight the differences in types of rooming houses. The first group lives in rooming houses near the relatively quiet parts of the Rough, mainly where the elderly poor reside. The dwellers in these types of rooming houses are relatively stable, well kept, and have little or no drug use and sex work. Individuals who live in these kinds of rooming house settings generally go to work when it is available, and within the context of the Rough, they live "decent" lives in attempting to earn money legally and stay off the streets. These rooming houses have singles as well as couples in them. Doll, a 30-year-old crack smoker, who recently moved into the rooming house market, described the house where she rents as quiet. She arrived in the Rough after having been steady-partner housed for what she described as "many years" with a drug dealer. In just six months she has been in several rooming houses and remains open to moving to one she perceives as better than her current room:

> I haven't been in the same one [rooming house]. I'm tryin' to find a better one. I pay sixty-five dollars a week—some places it might be more. It's pretty decent living. I never been in one that was like rowdy like that.

Individuals living in rooming houses like the one Doll described generally have low wage–paying, temporary, or underground jobs. Doll works at a body shop as a bookkeeper, but admits that she began turning tricks about a month prior to meeting me. Her clientele consists of a few regulars whose "visits" to her rooming house appear as if she has a few boyfriends coming by her room after leaving work. Right now, she believes she is the only one performing sex work in this house. In fact, several couples live in her rooming houses and pool their resources to remain a step above homelessness.

Gloria works in the temporary labor pool and finds herself changing rooming houses frequently. She admits that she sometimes misuses what little money she earns to buy drugs and doesn't have any money saved to make ends meet on the days she may not get picked for a job in the labor pool. Gloria attempted to explain the vicious cycle she faces.

> I'm working for tools and fools. It's not enough to really do anything but pay rent. Then after I pay rent, then I've got like fifteen, twenty dollars. I say, it's time to do something for myself. I done earned it. That just basically be that thought that be in my head. So go get me a couple of sacks, some beer and some cigarettes, and get me a bag of weed. Hey, I'm gonna party. Once that's gone, I still got my weed, and a few beers, and cigarettes. By the time I make it to somebody else's house, or they make it to my house, and it continues on. It's like a cycle. It keeps rolling and rolling and rolling.

Like Gloria, Sabrina works a low-wage job and tries to maintain a place to live off the streets. Despite her efforts to reduce the additional risks associated with being absolutely homeless, Sabrina describes how women in rooming houses can be displaced even if they are working and paying their rent. They rarely have written lease agreements. They do get a rent receipt from week to week, but they have very few rights as tenants. However, Sabrina received a notice from the rooming house owner that she would have to move within a month. In this case, the landlord informed them that he would be remodeling the house. In other cases, rooming house occupants are asked to move and are given no explanation. The house could have been sold to a new owner who may choose to convert it back to a single-family home and place it under Section 8, a government-sponsored housing program in which low-income participants get a voucher that pays a substantial portion of their rent. In fact, several Section 8 signs are placed in front of renovated homes throughout the Rough.

Despite their attempts to reduce risks associated with living literally on the streets, the rooming housed women face similar risk for HIV as their absolute homeless counterparts. The rooming housed women who work in the low wage–paying industry have somewhat of an advantage over the absolute homeless, as leaving the Rough for work each day allows them to have greater ties to mainstream society. Because some get a paycheck, the rooming housed may not put themselves at risk for HIV infection via unprotected sex with paying partners as often as do the absolute homeless. Nevertheless, when they are between jobs or out of money, they find themselves intermingling with the absolute homeless competing for sex work. The rooming housed women present a unique challenge for HIV prevention: There needs to be a clearly defined distinction between women who are in rooming houses and attempting to maintain a job and ties to their family, and those who are in rooming houses as sex workers. In addition, the motivation for change among women who are in rooming houses after having been evicted from apartments may differ tremendously from those who are moving up from absolute homelessness.

Michelle and Pamela's narratives highlight contrasting perspectives on what it is like to take risks within the context of living in a rooming house. First, Michelle became a rooming house renter for the purpose of performing sex work. Michelle's rooming house is occupied primarily by women who perform sex work, although non–sex workers live there as well. The key difference between her rooming house and a typical crack house is that she pays weekly rent to remain in her room, whereas crack house dwellers tend to pay for rooms by the hour and night. Crack house dwellers are "evicted" when they have no more money for drugs. This can be after a few hours or a few days. Rooming house renters are evicted when they have no money for rent.

Unlike Pamela who came to the Rough for homeownership, Michelle was lured to the Rough by a pimp to increase her clientele. She perceives herself to be an activist of sorts among crack-using prostitutes and often cautions them against "men who don't look right." According to Michelle, her motive is to drive up the price of sex work by stressing on the women to avoid bidding down for various sex requests. In addition, she attempts to work in groups with other women to avoid violent encounters with clientele who perceive the women to be tricking them out of their drugs and money. She admits that such approaches are hard because many of the women are on the streets and "strung out" and do not see the value of partnering with others.

Pamela, on the other hand, discussed how she became rooming housed after losing a single-family home she was purchasing in the Rough. She is a registered nurse who had to take a leave of absence for health reasons. During that time, Pamela's husband and her 22-year-old son attempted to pay the mortgage and support the drug habits of all three of these adult users. Over time, Pamela and her family were eight payments behind in the mortgage and eventually faced a foreclosure. At this time, Pamela and her husband moved into a rooming house. She reminded me of just how close her rooming house is to the one she was purchasing. "You remember where you saw me sitting on the porch. That was my house. Now I'm in the rooming house next door. Ain't no way I can get it back."

As one who had typically maintained a lower middle-class lifestyle even as a drug user, Pamela expressed frustration toward rooming house living. She and her husband didn't understand the "unwritten rules" associated with the rooming house, one of which is the need to have someone watch your room when you are working or away for extended periods. This resulted in having their valuables stolen. I asked Pamela, "What's the biggest problem you are dealing with right now?" As did so many other women in the study, Pamela emotionally responded, "Housing, housing, housing!" We discussed her strategy for dealing with her dilemma, and she asserted that she and her husband are saving all the money they can for an apartment. According to Pamela, "the little money my husband make—he don't make a whole lot either and he's putting it back so that we can get us another place. So, hopefully in the next two weeks we will have something."

Pamela actually brightened up as she discussed her preparations for moving out of the rooming house. "For the last six weeks [my husband] been working down at the Apparel Mart. We got some nice stuff to go into the apartment when we do get it. They gave us some dishes and some other items. Then a friend of ours gave us a dinette set. So I done been down and come up to what I had. Now I'm back down, but I'm slowly coming back up and I'm going to keep on keeping on."

Pamela reinforces the idea that rooming houses are a middle ground between homeless and apartment living. For some women, this becomes a critical time to make agency choices concerning their willingness to take the necessary steps to avoid slipping into homelessness. At the same time, there are structural factors that must be examined in analyzing one's willingness and ability to move toward permanent housing verses homelessness. For example, Pamela's husband is a "day labor" landscaper, which means that he works when the weather is good and when contractors pick him. When he is between jobs, there is no unemployment compensation. Even when working, there are no benefits, such as health care, worker's compensation, or retirement—benefits that even full-time employed mainstream Americans who do not use drugs grapple with not having, as the political economy is structured to "benefit" big corporations.

HOUSE WOMEN

The major distinction between house women and street women is that house women have the privilege of more permanent housing relative to their street counterparts. However, beyond that they have several differences that can be explained via a conceptual framework that places house women in one of three categories: (1) the heads of household, (2) the family housed, or (3) the steady-partner housed. House women have access to more stable resources relative to street women, as well as social support from extended family members. From an individual standpoint, many house women acknowledge that they participate in "street-like" behavior, yet structurally they have access to housing that serves as an option to lower high-risk behavior. In fact, the average house woman has been in her dwelling for at least four years, and many of the family housed never left home to begin with.

The Heads of Household

The heads of household are women (nine) who live in apartments or houses where they are legally and financially responsible for the property they occupy. Overall, the heads of household are the most stable of all the women in this study. They are subdivided into two categories of subsidized and nonsubsidized renters. The two subsidized heads of household (Corie and Shanté) are in the Section 8 government housing program. The other seven women are nonsubsidized and pay market rent for their apartments. Three of the women (Martha, Peaches, and Karen) get disability checks, and another three (Frankie, Lisa, and Shanté) receive welfare checks and are caring for minor children. Four of the women (Frankie, Shanté, Lisa, and Martha) have partners that live with them.

The heads of household women may find themselves facing similar dilemmas of locating new housing arrangements as do rooming housed women. Peaches lived in a set of apartments that was condemned and was notified that she had thirty days to vacate. She was able to find a new place across the street; however, many women in her apartment complex became street women as they scrambled for new housing. As poor heads of household, Frankie and Shanté are at the mercy of social workers who decide whether or not they remain eligible for government benefits. Both have been notified that their eligibility for welfare is up in a few months, at which time they may face a change of status from heads of household, depending on what resources are available to them. Many of the women who are now hustling homeless and rooming housed were once heads of household, but were displaced during the dismantling of housing projects and welfare "as we know it."

Like other women in the Rough, if Frankie and Shanté cannot find jobs prior to their eligibility ending for welfare, they may engage in illegal behavior to make ends meet. Both are high school dropouts with limited work experience. Frankie confided that she already sells sex in order to get drugs, and avoids taking money from the household to purchase crack. However, if she loses her welfare benefits, she may increase her participation in the sex trade for additional money to support her family and drug habit. Shanté, on the other hand, may decide to intensify her current part-time drug-dealing efforts. Other heads of household women who supplement their social service income include Lisa, who works at a fast food restaurant; Corie, who is paid "under the table" as an orderly; Martha, who charges street women (and men) to smoke crack inside her apartment; and Peaches, who rents out a room in her house by the hour to sex workers.

There are four heads of household women who have live-in partners, but maintain that these men are not the primary breadwinners. Frankie, Shanté, Lisa, and Martha all have partners who contribute financially to the household. Frankie discussed getting into constant fights with her partner because he suspects that she prostitutes herself. Shanté is frustrated because her mate, who is a drug dealer, is constantly on the corner with other women. Shanté claims that she is no longer having sex with her steady partner. She describes why she stopped having sex with him.

> We don't even be intimate no more like we used to 'cause I don't know what he be doing out there. Sometime he'll stay gone. I don't even hardly just trust being intimate with him. 'Cause I know that's how a man gone be.

Later, however, Shanté confided that she had been in the hospital a week prior to my interview with her, diagnosed with a tubal pregnancy. Even if the baby was not her steady partner's, clearly Shanté has unprotected sex, and her perception of herself as a low risk taker may be inaccurate.

Lisa's narrative is typical of the dilemmas facing low-income head of household women. She lives in a low-income apartment community and receives $330 per month from welfare for three children. In addition she gets another $400 in food stamps. Her most recent job was at a fast food restaurant; however, she is now in between jobs, as she is caring for her son who had brain surgery to remove a tumor. The social worker at the children's hospital assessed her apartment to be an unfit environment for her son to recover. Lisa's mother, who lives in the suburban house where she grew up, was able to accommodate the sick child; however, the other two boys remain in Lisa's custody in the apartment labeled unfit for the older boy to heal. The social worker from the hospital assisted in helping her to move to the top of the Section 8 list for subsidized housing.

Lisa has been in her current apartment for three years and on and off welfare for almost twelve years. Her rent is $310. She describes how she recently had to get her mother to document family support in order to remain on welfare, after her case officer began questioning how Lisa was making up the difference to cover her household expense.

> They were gonna try to cut me off if I didn't give them some kind of documentation saying how I was paying these other bills when my rent is three hundred and ten dollars and the check was nothing but three hundred and thirty dollars. So I went to her and she said, "well you got to show me some kind of letter or something from your parents, your friends, somebody who making up these other bills." And you know like, I'm going to tell you to be quite honest. Then they gave me three hundred and thirty dollars. I took three hundred and ten dollars of that and paid my rent, 'cause I always need somewhere to stay. The rest of it, I'll make it like I make it. I'll make it even if I have to go to friends, family, boyfriends, cousins, whoever. And then she told me, she say, "we going to discontinue you if you don't show us some kind of proof of how you making up this difference." So I went to my mom, which was lucky, because she had helped me pay my light bill and help me do that when I was on the welfare and wasn't working. So I went to my mom. I told my mom, "Look, these people trying to cut my stuff off. Write a letter stating that you been helping me pay this light bill and this and this and that." So she wrote the letter and I took it to the lady and they looked at it and she realized, I guess she looked at it and said, this ain't her handwriting, so okay it must be all right.

The caseworker was probably indicating that Lisa had a man living with her. In the seventies the government conducted midnight "panty raids" to find men living with women who received welfare checks. However, today caseworkers try to get the same information by inquiring about the women's household expenses in comparison to income. In fact, Lisa did have a steady partner living with her for a period of time. Lisa discussed feeling depressed as she was readjusting after her boyfriend moved out without notice. They dated almost two years and had an 11-month-old son together. According to Lisa, he contributed to the household income, as he worked as a heating and air conditioning technician. I asked Lisa about her partner, and at first she stated that she "kicked him to the curb." When I asked her to tell me what happened, she retracted her story and admitted that he just "up and left." Now, Lisa finds herself having to date again after believing she would be in this relationship for some time, because it was a man she reunited with after having dated him earlier when she was in high school.

Lisa recalled having a little anxiety when she took the HIV test earlier because even though she knew she had been faithful to her partner, she questioned his faithfulness. According to Lisa, "It's not all the time who you messing with. You may be messing with somebody and they be messing with somebody else and the cycle goes on and on and on." She went on to describe how she attempts to minimize her risks.

> I just go in my house. I get mine (crack cocaine) and go in my house. I try to keep us a substantial amount of money. I don't never make myself run completely out of money. I'll try to keep a couple of dollars here, a couple of dollars there, somewhere. My mind as a person still there, but I don't let it control my whole mind. That why I said I'm able to maintain my house, pay my rent, keep my children. I can't go to my family 'cause they will be looking at me like, "you couldn't be one of ours." I don't be out there. After dark I be in my house 'cause I got kids. Sometime I would look out my window. You can see girls walking down the streets and men stopping in cars. I don't know what it is about this street, but they love it. You can see girls—they jump in cars. And that worries me too, because when you jump in a car we may not never see you again. That's they lifestyle, but that's not me. I got children. I can't be out there running up and down the street after dark.

The key characteristics of the heads of households are they have a place to live and a safer place to smoke crack, which may reduce their risk for HIV. In addition, having custody of their children and having to care for them daily puts parameters and constraints on these women that reduce their risk. However, several have steady partners that are "in and out" of their lives, which adds to their risk for infection. Also, these women's desire to hide their behavior from their mainstream family members may limit social support that could result in heightened risks as they search for ways to tide themselves over until the next month when some receive welfare or disability checks. It is precisely at these times when even the relatively stable heads of household women may find themselves briefly exhibiting the risky behavior often associated with street women.

The Family Housed

The family-housed women live with a family member, usually their mothers. Some live with grandmothers and aunts. Many have never left home in the first place. The commonality is that they have housing in the Rough due to a close relative's generosity. While the women in this category have a permanent residence, many take to the streets and can often be seen in the Rough interacting with the hustling homeless. In fact, the main difference between the family-housed women and the hustling homeless is that the family housed have maintained their living arrangements and take advantage of their opportunities to sleep, eat, and bath at home on a regular basis. The hustling homeless, on the other hand, acknowledge that they "can go home," but choose to remain on the streets for extended periods of time. The family housed, then, share a lot in common with the hustling homeless in terms of their lifestyle of sex work and drug use in crack houses. However, the family-housed women believe they are different from the hustling homeless because they do not stay away from home as long, and they take advantage of offers to remain socially insulated with their family.

Sonya recalls how she once was a hustling homeless, but by the time she came to the HIP House, she had recently given birth to a baby girl and reclassified herself as a "family-girl." According to Sonya, "I wasn't out on the streets but I was more like coming out of the streets when I found out about it [the HIP House]. Jumpin' in and out of cars and I was messin' 'round with different guys."

This group's vulnerability is rooted in having to find alternative locations for their sex and drug activities. Because some are members of families who will not allow them to do drugs in the house, many find themselves interacting with "full-time" street women. In addition, most of the family-housed women in this study are unemployed and thus depend on sex work and other hustles as a means of self-support. The only feature that separates them from full-time street women is that they have a home to go to once they have smoked their crack. However, in reality, many family-housed women describe themselves as getting caught up in the streets or crack houses and often remain away from the family house for extended periods of time, ranging from one night to a week.

If the women could leave crack-smoking scenes and return home once they have done drugs, then in the absolute they are not at risk for HIV/AIDS. However, instead of returning home, some begin to participate in sex work to maintain on the streets a little longer. This is the critical point when family-housed women begin to place themselves at risk for HIV/AIDS. Mattie tries to provide her family-housed daughters who use crack with the option to smoke at home as a way to help them avoid becoming temporary street women. Mattie explains, "When I found out that they were doing it [crack cocaine], I told them I'd rather you do it at home than to do it out there in the street with anybody and anything."

Overall, the family housed are at risk because some prefer to remain in the streets even when their families insist on providing them a safety net. Others may be temporarily dismissed from the home for something as minor as stealing food, or as major as taking drugs or money from others in the household. During these adult "time-outs" these women take to the street and often exhibit the behaviors typically associated with "street women," even if for shorter periods of time. In the end, however, these women are allowed to return home, as they have mothers like Mattie, who simply don't want to see their daughters in the street.

The Steady-Partner Housed

The steady-partner housed women depend on their significant others for housing. These couples may share a rooming house or pay market rent for an apartment. Four of the women live in an apartment, one lives in a house, and four live in a rooming house. What separates this group of women from others who may also live with a steady partner is that the women in this group acknowledge they only have a steady place to live because of the income from their partners. Other women in the study have steady partners that live with them. However, partners of the steady-partner housed are considered the primary breadwinners. The steady-partner housed women discuss their daily routines as similar to that of any other working-class couple. These women describe themselves as housewives who cook and clean. Only one has a teenager who lives with her. The others have adult children, or adolescents who live with other family members.

The steady-partner housed women's significant others have jobs ranging from day laborers (four) to a drug dealer and a hustler. Another one is retired from the army and now owns rooming houses. There were two women who did not mention the occupation or means of income for their steady partners.

These women have steady partners with very different patterns in terms of drugs and alcohol use. Tomeka and Ingrid claim their partners are drug and alcohol free. Both reported being abused by their partners because of the women's drug use. Lois, Allison, and Dee-Dee have partners who drink alcohol, but do not use drugs. All three of them are able to smoke at home, despite their partner's dislike of their drug use. Carmen and Punkin have partners who use drugs and drink alcohol, with Carmen's partner of thirty-one years also being an injection drug user. Both of these women hustle with their partners for drug money.

Five of the steady-partner housed are sex workers. Four of the five expressed that they have regular customers who also are married. Allison prides herself on being a lucky gambler as a main source of income, but has about twelve customers whom she describes as "older married men." She has a girlfriend who lives some five miles from the Rough. Allison pays the girlfriend ten dollars per customer to allow her to use a room in her house to perform sex work. According to Allison, her partner "Leroy" suspects that she is selling her body, but is not sure.

Many of the women echoed this type of suspicion among their partners. I pushed back several times and suggested that these partners know they are sex workers. In fact, I challenged some by asking if I could talk to the men myself. I had no intentions of doing so, but I just wanted to know what they thought their partners' perspectives were of their drug and sex behavior. Allison commented that I would have to catch Leroy when he is sober, but she warned that he would say some bad things about her. I asked how bad and to that she replied, "He will say some bad stuff, like she sell plenty pussy and I know she do. He will have the worsest things in the world to say about me. But he'll kill a rock about me."

While street women experienced more street violence, seven women in this group of house women discussed domestic violence as central to their relationships. Most did not describe themselves as victims, and generally attributed their partners' violent behavior as a "natural" reaction to their own drug use. Tomeka explains, "He doesn't do drugs or drink. He can tell when I hit that shit. That's when he dog me. Otherwise he don't bother me." Ingrid's account of turmoil due to her drugs was milder in that she says they "fuss all the time" because he doesn't know that she goes through with drugs.

Perhaps the closest I came to understanding the impact of domestic violence in these women's lives was through my interaction with Cynthia. I was her interventionist and she talked for about forty-five minutes of being tired of the fighting. The very next session, the outreach worker brought her in beat up and bleeding. I looked at her and she looked at me. Without exchanging a word, I began administering first aid. I told her we could always reschedule. She wanted to move forward with her session. It couldn't have been for the money because this was session number two. She would not be paid again until her last session. Initially, I felt guilty that I had somehow talked to her about self-empowerment in a way that may have triggered this type of violent reaction. In the end, I believed that this was a violent man who would kill her to show he had the power in their relationship. However, this time I kept quiet, because I had read that abused women's problems worsen if they try to leave.

Punkin described how the constant bickering and fighting often leads to her becoming a "temporary street woman" until tensions cool down at home. She explained,

> It's because of him that I'm out there. He don't send me out there to turn tricks. We just get into a fight or something. He know what that consists of. I rather stay outside and run the streets than to go get stuck up in one of them folk crack house.

The steady-partner housed pride themselves on being able to maintain a relationship, and portray some aspects of traditional living in their everyday lives. Almost all (eight) described themselves as "loners" who smoked their drugs at home. They distinguished themselves from street women by stating that they don't have to be out on the streets. They sincerely believe that street women are jealous of them because they have a steady partner who provides them a place to live. Punkin, who admits that her partner was responsible for the pins she had in her jaw a few months prior to her interview, explained, "They jealous of me because I'm with him and don't even have to be out on the street."

These women discussed their perceptions of their steady partner's faithfulness. Dee-Dee, for example, believes her husband is propositioned by the women on the street, but that he is too stingy with his money to pay for sex. She jokingly stated that if they pay him for it, perhaps he will have sex with them, but he is not going to give them any money. Carmen, who has been with Mark for thirty-one years, says that she doesn't have the desire to have sex, so he doesn't either. On the other hand, Punkin, who is HIV positive, believes that her partner infected her.

Lois explains that she has taken her bill money and spent it on drugs in the past. She says that her husband has often paid the bills to maintain their household. She describes her husband as one who supports her and loves her even though she smokes crack.

> Half the time I had my own money. Or I would buy my drugs on what they call breakdown—sell some and smoke some. So, I always had me some money and my husband always was there for me. He told me "I will go buy it for you." I thank God that he stuck by me.

Lois had confided to her interventionist at the HIP House that she had slept with men for money and drugs in very desperate moments. I found this out when I reviewed her HIP file after interviewing her. I was confused and a little hurt that Lois did not share that information with me. Lois really fooled me. Somehow I thought she was different from the other women I had met. She looks great. She works. She maintains a household. She goes to church. I guess she wanted to put her best foot forward and provide a positive image since she stopped doing drugs. I wish I had known to ask more about her sex life outside her marriage. In analyzing my notes and transcripts, I realize that Lois had given me the opportunity to probe more. She said, "*Half the time* I have my own money." I should have asked about what she did *the other half of the time* when she did not have any money.

Lois was adamant in stating "I never been a street person. Never have and never will." She talked about a time when her husband actually came to the house where she bought and smoked drugs to confront her. According to Lois, several of the men defended her by telling him that she doesn't have sex with anyone in the house. She admits that her method is to try to "con" them out of drugs by talking sexy and by looking and smelling good. However, as she shared with her interventionist, conning did not always work and sometimes resulted in exchanging sex for drugs or money.

As Punkin succinctly suggests, however, women who share a home with steady partners can and often do reach points of desperation. Apparently, Lois is not exempt. While she chose not to discuss what happens the times she does not have her own money, it is clear that steady partner housed women sometimes take on characteristics typically attributed to street women in order to maintain their drug use habits. According to Punkin, "When we broke we all jump in cars!"

Perhaps the commonality among the steady partnered in terms of their risk for HIV is that they rarely use condoms with this person, even though most women are suspicious that their partner cheats. The pool of "decent" eligible bachelors in urban poor ghettos is so limited that those women who do manage to find a steady partner feel privileged in such a setting. Thus, she may tolerate a "man being a man" if it results in her maintaining her status as a kept woman in this environment. In addition, these women often change steady partners. During the times they are between partners some may face a heightened risk for HIV infection. Others, however, may protect themselves and only stop using condoms when the relationship approaches monogamy.

While the women discussed their risks for HIV intervention within the context of their current living conditions, it is important to note that these drug-using women generally change housing types more often than do the non–drug-using poor. The street women in particular discussed changing housing more frequently. Most were homeless for less than six months with the exception of Mona, who was homeless for nine years. Clearly, the absolute homeless arrived at such a state after losing more permanent housing. In like manner, the hustling homeless are constantly "in between living arrangements." For example, they may have a rooming house for a month, live with family for a short time, and then move closer to appearing absolute homeless for some period.

The house women in this study described being in their living arrangements anywhere from three months to eleven years. The average length of time for a house woman in one type of housing is four years. The heads of household are the most stable and the steady partnered are the least stable in terms of housing arrangements. While I have chosen to analyze the women during a point in time in terms of their housing, an in-depth analysis of how women are at risk as they transition up or down the spectrum of housing types could prove helpful in future interventions.

In this chapter, I have presented risk factors for HIV as grounded in the women's narratives concerning their housing arrangements. These women's perceptions about the neighborhood have great implications for the future planning and implementation of HIV/AIDS prevention programs in high-risk environments. Prevention programmers must think critically about daily realities of lives of at-risk women. In the past decade several ethnographers have provided rich detail about other Rough places in urban America that serve as insiders' perspectives in helping HIV prevention interventionists contextualize the social and economic dimensions associated with risk in poor urban areas. To varying degrees they address the HIV and crack cocaine epidemics plaguing urban communities. However, none approach these social problems within the context of attempting to change one's risk factors in an urban ghetto where drug use and risky sex have become the norm.

While providing an extensive account of urban ethnographies is beyond the scope of this study, it is important to note that collectively, these researchers provide a comprehensive body of literature on the ways in which various social problems impact the drug-using and non–drug-using poor alike. For example, disinvestment (Bach and West, 1993), institutional racism (Wilson, 1996; Holzier, 1995), lack of affordable housing (Bartelt, 1993), drugs (Sterk, 1999; Dash, 1996; Bourgois, 1995), patriarchy (Edin and Lein, 1997; Fine and Weis,

1997), and the loss of living wage jobs (Wilson, 1996; MacCleod, 1995; Bartlett, 1993) are just a few of the social issues that affect the majority of urban poor dwellers. These urban studies assert that inner-city communities over the past decade have witnessed a rise in an urban underclass and decline of socially organized inner-city minority communities (Tross, 2001; Cummings, 1998; Wilson, 1996). Several link their description of ghetto poor communities to a larger perspective centered on deindustrialization, with decreased job opportunities for poorly educated men and women of color (Newman, 1999). They further argue that a key consequence of a failing replacement economic strategy for urban areas after disinvestment resulted in concentrated unemployment, with many opting to participate in the informal economy that features illicit, as well as legal—but unstable—jobs (Bourgois, 1995; Fagan, 1993; Kirschenman and Neckerman, 1991). For example, several women in this study work seasonally as ticket takers and food servers at the various sports stadiums near the Rough. However, during the off season, there is no formal assistance to help them manage.

My work builds on existing studies on urban poor dwellers by giving voice to poor women often treated as a homogeneous group in leading urban ethnographies. For example, Anderson (1999) described high-risk environments and high-risk behavior in terms of the drugs, violence, and street crime that appear to be heightened in more alienated parts of the ghetto. He suggested that even within high-risk environments, one could observe decent families trying to maintain and adhere to mainstream values of hard work. It is the street families, as he observed them, who participate in high-risk behavior. He termed their actions "loose behavior" as characterized by violence, drug use, teen pregnancy, welfare scams, staying out very late, and underground economy rackets. In an earlier work, Anderson (1990) described the drug culture and the direct ways in which those who use drugs may be at risk for HIV/AIDS as follows:

> Dealers tend to have certain corners and spaces "served up," marked off as their own territory, and may prevent other dealers from selling either at a particular corner or even in the general area. . . . Addicts may gravitate to a crack house, usually a non-descript dwelling where drugs are easily purchased. . . . Some

women wear no underwear prepared to engage in all types of sexual acts in exchange for drugs. They eventually leave the place not with money, but with a number of highs to their credit. Sex is sold for the pleasure of the drug not to make a living, as was common in the past. (p. 85)

While I consider Anderson's work to be an extremely significant contribution in the field of urban ethnography, my research contrasts his findings in that I observed both street and decent families in urban poor neighborhoods grappling with risky sex and drug behaviors that place both types of families at risk for HIV. The major difference is street families are more visible and easily observed during participant observation. However, because of the state of the political economy within poor communities, members of decent families find themselves participating in behaviors Anderson reserves for "street families." Families with more permanent housing and relatively stable ties to mainstream society may not be as visible as are their street counterparts, yet they are still engaging in risky behavior that leaves them vulnerable to the spread of HIV/AIDS.

I have attempted to link the problems of the women in this study to those faced by the non–drug-using poor. The crisis of homelessness and affordable housing are issues for urban poor throughout America. Moreover, many individuals grapple with belonging to several underprivileged subgroups, causing some to face multiple oppressions of poverty, domestic violence, and gender and race discrimination. Contextually, with the onset of crack cocaine and the spread of HIV, the urban ghetto has become a place where marginalized women become even more marginal. This devastating consequence of poverty is due primarily to the scramble among the publicly labeled "deserving and undeserving" poor for scarce social service resources. One team of seemingly frustrated ethnographers (Crane, Quirk, and van der Straten, 2002) best summed up the dilemma facing the urban poor when they concluded,

It became clear through the course of our study that many participating couples were living in a world in which a positive HIV antibody test or an AIDS diagnosis could result in an improved quality of life by allowing for increased access to Supplemental Security Income, subsidized housing, food and services. This situation is in part a consequence of recent policy decisions related to the "War on Drugs" and welfare reform. These policies have contributed to the creation of an economy of poverty in which the sick, needy, and addicted must compete against each other for scarce resources. Within such an economy, an HIV or AIDS diagnosis may actually operate as a commodity.

The women helped me understand the black feminization of Crane and associates' (2002) argument. For poor African-American women—especially those who have been deleted from welfare, public housing, food stamps, and Medicaid—becoming HIV positive may be the best way to regain these resources. As Johnsie explained it, "People are not dying from AIDS, they are living with HIV." In addition, given the sex-ratio imbalance among urban poor women and men, how do you explain to a woman who has been married to the same man for thirty-one years that because her husband injects drugs and is in and out of jail for petty crimes that she should insist he use condoms?

Only after contextualizing such risks as relative to one's reality did my personal frustrations of seeing the women continuing to engage in risky behavior subside. These realities are engrained mentally and structurally in the lives of these women and must be considered by those who implement prevention intervention programs. Therefore, a clear understanding of how these African-American women live and take risks in the Rough is key to understanding how to more effectively deliver prevention intervention strategies that meet the needs of this target population.

PRINCIPLES TO GUIDE HIV PREVENTION INITIATIVES BASED ON WOMEN'S LIVING ARRANGEMENTS

Existing HIV prevention programs can be strengthened by developing modules and strategies that acknowledge that differences in living arrangements impact one's risk for HIV (Downing et al., 1999). For example, the absolute homeless are often plagued with other issues, including being clinically diagnosed as mentally ill and trying to avoid facing felony charges. Others who are absolute homeless simply have lost permanent housing due to changes in the economy, domestic violence, drug use, or cuts in social services. Community-based HIV prevention interventions can focus on setting short-term goals, known as "small wins," that lower risk within the context of these larger structural constraints (Gentry, Elifson, and Sterk, 2005).

The hustling homeless are characterized by frequent trips to jail for misdemeanors. Perhaps these typical thirty- to ninety-day sentences may serve as the most appropriate time to link them to community-based services that specialize in reaching this "hard to track" group (Wexler et al., 1994). HIV prevention counselors working with women living in rooming houses need to determine if a client is moving up from the streets or spiraling down from having more permanent housing. In essence, those moving up to better living arrangements may be motivated to make even more positive changes. On the other hand, if a client is in a rooming house because she lost more stable living arrangements, behavioral risk reduction may not be seen as a priority for her (Gentry, Elifson, and Sterk, 2005).

HIV prevention providers who work with women with more permanent housing must partner with less stigmatizing collaborative partners. For example, unlike street women, women with housing are more likely to interface with pediatricians, personal care doctors, faith-based staff, trusted family members, and child care providers. Because women with relatively stable housing perceive themselves to have more in common with mainstream organizations and individuals, HIV prevention messages targeting this group will be more effective if delivered in less stigmatizing agencies. Women who live with family members may need special assistance in leaving their home environment as a first step in lowering their risk behavior, particularly if others in the home continue to do drugs and practice unsafe sex. Still others are in families in which family interventions may be more appropriate, as there may be multiple family members at risk for HIV infection. Finally, the women who live with steady partners may be better served in HIV prevention programs that target intimate couples with respect and value for marginalized individuals in relationships. Specific approaches to address the needs of high-risk couples are discussed in Chapter 6, which deals with the women's risk in intimate partner relationships (Gentry, Elifson, and Sterk, 2005).

Chapter 3

Rough Family Relations

I can go over my family house for six months and don't smoke dope. Once I hit [the Rough], I'm smoking crack again. I can stay a month over mama house or my sister's and don't have no desire, but once I hit Simpson Road the desire of drugs come back. You got to go where people are going to work everyday. People that's going to church. People that care for you; that don't have no nonsense in their house. That's the only way you gone get yourself off drugs.

Allison, a 40-year-old crack user and sex worker

In Allison's account of her own family relations, she suggests that black families of orientation have been underutilized as a source of strength in helping women achieve their HIV prevention goals. As I mentioned in the introduction, one of the most perplexing issues is that of so many girls from seemingly "good families" ending up in the Rough. As such, I had very strong feelings in analyzing and drafting this chapter on women's familial relationships. While I have had the privilege to study and teach family studies as a scholar and researcher, nothing prepared me for the feelings that surfaced about my own vulnerabilities as a high-risk youth who lived on the edge of an invisible thin line in the black community that is thought to separate decent and street families. As these women suggest, families of orientation over the life course can be a source of strength and resilience even with limited economic resources, while simultaneously subjecting one to stresses and strains that may ultimately increase one's risk for HIV infection.

Black Women's Risk for HIV: Rough Living
© 2007 by The Haworth Press, Taylor & Francis Group. All rights reserved.
doi:10.1300/5784_03

The black feminist theme of the unique experiences of African-American women guided the inquiry into the women's family relationships as I asked myself, "What does it mean to be a high-risk woman socialized in a black family?" In essence, how does the role of daughter and sister serve as risk and protection for black women? What does it mean to be labeled high risk as a young black girl in either a decent or street family setting? In asking these questions from a black feminist perspective, I hoped to discover a hidden dimension of family life that can be used to inform the development of family-centered interventions in the lives of high-risk women.

Family systems perspectives have emerged as a dominant theme in HIV/AIDS literature with family-centered programs designed to help HIV/AIDS-infected individuals cope through various stages of disease management (Reeves, Merriam, and Courtenay, 1999). In comparison, HIV prevention research has not fully articulated evidence-based roles for families in HIV prevention in the lives of high-risk women (Gilbert and Wright, 2003). However, HIV prevention for women in general overlooks family systems with most programs implemented using individualistic approaches to behavioral change (Auerback and Coates, 2000; Bandura, 1994).

In examining family of orientation as defined as the family one is either born or adopted into, I draw heavily on family sociological perspectives of the family as a group of people who live together and provide economic and emotional support for all of its members (Benokraitis, 1999). However, in examining high-risk youth outcomes, studies tend to focus on the correlation between family income and risk factors (Boyd, 1993). My analysis of women's accounts of their families suggest that measurements of economic well-being also must include variables that are more gendered in nuance such as emotional support and sexual molestation. Their accounts of family relations support the idea that future HIV prevention interventions should take into account the gender differences associated with growing up in either a decent or street family. As such, this chapter explores women's past and present relationships with one or both of their biological parents.

My advocacy for families of orientation as a source of strength in HIV prevention is grounded in an encounter I had with Gayle. Gayle arrived at the HIP House each week almost like clockwork on Friday afternoons. She had graduated and completed her six-month follow-up;

however, program graduates were allowed to return to the HIP House for condoms, food, and clothing even after their sessions ended. While the staff regulated the goings and comings of graduates, we were all a bit lenient in providing food and were even more generous toward women who were pregnant. As Gayle was pregnant and in a domestically violent relationship during this particular time, she was at the HIP House almost daily and would be patient until one of us was free to assist her with meals and any kind of counseling we could provide between scheduled sessions. She often complemented me on my outfits and reminisced about the times she used to dress nice. She often complained about the pressure she was under in her current relationship and how horrible some of the recent fights had been since she wasn't able to turn dates to supply their drug habit while she was pregnant.

As I interacted with Gayle, I couldn't help but think about my own family of orientation and how they might react to me if I were a crack user. As a black woman with extended family support, I concluded that they would intervene and try to get me some help. I also know that even though they may have the desire to help me, they are clueless as to the most effective methods and approaches for doing so. I sincerely believed that these women's families would be eager to do the same for their daughters and sisters if only they knew what to do and had some guidance on how to do it. As I thought about how my own mother would want to help me, one day I got up the nerve to ask Gayle if her mother knew she was a crack user and living in the Rough. She assured me that her mother knew of her whereabouts. At the end of the short conversation, Gayle gave me her mother's telephone number, and I called her the same evening. I introduced myself and she explained in a very saddened tone that she had driven through the Rough earlier in the week and she said, "It hurt me to my heart to see my child on that corner with those raggedy clothes and her hair all matted to her head." She further explained that she doesn't know how her daughter got into this predicament because she raised her to dress nice and she was active in school. She said after graduating from high school, she kept a good job and took good care of her child. She begged me to try to help her daughter get into treatment so she wouldn't deliver a baby addicted to crack cocaine. A few days later, Gayle came into the HIP House grinning from ear to ear and gave me a big hug. She announced to everyone in the HIP House, "My friend here called my mama on me. I didn't know ya'll cared like that!" The fact that Gayle interpreted my calling her mother as an act of "caring" suggests that there is promise in developing HIV prevention models that include modules for strengthening and or building on family relations.

Other stories similar to the interaction between Gayle and myself convinced me that the role of families of orientation have been underexplored in HIV prevention research as motivators and barriers among high-risk women. As I read the women's accounts of their families of orientation, I couldn't help but wonder if the black community has overexaggerated the strength and resilience of the black family when it comes to steering youth away from drug abuse and high-risk sex. Black women need to understand how their family relationships impact their ability and willingness to address the behaviors that place them at risk for HIV infection.

To be clear, there is much in the literature on family interventions for youth at risk for HIV, most of which centers on abstinence from sex (Dittus et al., 2004; CDC, 2002). However, the literature lacks HIV prevention programs that focus on reconnecting black women to their families of orientation. A starting point for developing such a model that can be added to existing HIV prevention programs for enhanced effectiveness is to examine high-risk women's accounts of their family relationships. The first part of this analysis on families of orientation focuses on the structural dimensions of the family, highlighting primarily socioeconomic well-being. I draw heavily from Anderson's (1999) work *Code of the Street* in which he discussed street and decent families in an inner-city setting. Theoretically, I apply black feminist perspectives to tease out risks and resilience as girls face risks across class lines that may go underexplored when applying existing conceptual frameworks for examining family relationships.

GROWING UP DECENT

There were twenty-eight women who defined themselves as having grown up in decent families they described as fully integrated into mainstream society. The term "fully integrated" in this case refers to adhering to American values toward education, employment, and norms of abstinence from sex and drugs for the family's adolescents. Decent families, according to these women, reflect being reared in a home where parents worked to achieve the American Dream of homeownership, retired from living wage–paying jobs, and raised children to be good community citizens with the expectation that they will ultimately do better educationally and economically than their parents.

While most of the women describing their family upbringing as "decent" recalled having both biological parents in the household in the early years, several discussed experiencing parental separations and divorce. Still others described how stepfathers entered their lives ranging anywhere from when they were toddlers to teenagers. The women who grew up in "decent families" were more likely to characterize their neighborhoods and homes as positive and supportive environments for raising children. In fact, women from decent families often pointed to their own choices and behaviors, primarily in their teenage years, as turning points for engaging in drug selling and using, either with a boyfriend or with peers. For example, Tracie describes how both of her parents exhausted themselves and their economic resources to steer her in the right direction. However, according to Tracie, her parents were no match for the school and community environments where she succumbed to drug use and hanging out with other youth whose parents were less strict. She says her parents even threatened her as a last resort to try to get her to change her behavior.

> I was an honor student. My mother and father had big plans for me once I finished school. Either go to college or go in the service. It was gonna be one or the other. But when I went into senior high school, there were drugs. Messing with the boys and hanging on the corners and cutting classes and smoking the weed. They [my family] saw it coming and they tried to stop me. They tried to warn me. They'd threaten. That didn't do no good.

As is typical among mainstream black families, Tracie's parents attempted to protect her from the risk behaviors commonly associated with dysfunctional and pathological families. In fact, prior to the crack cocaine epidemic, decent families safely assumed their role was to help their black girls avoid teen pregnancy. However, as the crack cocaine problem initially was socially constructed as an inner-city phenomenon, many decent families simply were unaware of the level of exposure their children had to this devastating drug. As Tracie confirms, it was the school environment where she was introduced to the dangers of crack cocaine, and not in her home.

Daisy, a 41-year-old, has positive memories of growing up in a family where her father was a hardworking entrepreneur. Daisy was an avid athlete and went to college on a basketball scholarship. She asserts that after successfully transitioning from an adolescent in the Rough during the 1970s, when it was primarily a thriving black middle-class area, she tried drugs for the first time on a college campus in rural Georgia. According to Daisy, her weekly routine growing up mirrored that of a typical stable middle-class family, including high levels of school involvement, participation in team sports and religious activities, as well as working a part-time job.

Portia arrived in Atlanta as a teenager when her mother, who is a social worker and professor, moved to the area to take a job at a local university. Portia remembered growing up in the suburbs of New Jersey, where she and her brother were adopted into a home and she recalls having opportunities and material possessions generally associated with the American middle class in general. According to Portia, "I got everything I wanted. I had four dollhouses. I was spoiled rotten. My mother worked in New York and we lived in Jersey in Red Bank. I had the best life. I don't know what in the hell happened!" Portia's mother attempted to raise her adopted children in an environment away from drug use and prostitution. However, as Portia described, parents can overcompensate with material gifts and lack of discipline. Also, Portia was old enough to know she was adopted and never felt she fit in with the other middle-class girls in the neighborhood. She remembered feeling more comfortable and accepted by the kids from her old neighborhood, and as soon as she was old enough to use public transportation, she began living between both worlds, and ultimately found herself spending more time in the inner cities of New York and New Jersey rather than in her middle-class suburban neighborhood. Once in Atlanta a few years later, Portia made her way to the inner city, where again she began interacting with what she referred to as "the wrong crowd." This time her interaction escalated to another level as she became intimately involved with a local drug dealer and soon gave birth to the first of three children. According to Portia, she lived a

"New Jack" lifestyle for a few years before her partner went to jail for drug distribution.

Cynthia, a 42-year-old, grew up in a suburb of Miami. Like Portia, Cynthia enjoyed the economic security of a middle-class upbringing. However, unlike Portia, who lacked discipline and punishment for her failure to comply with parental rules, Cynthia's home life was much stricter. In fact, she ran away at fourteen to escape the physical punishment from a strict father who demanded that she be home each evening before the streetlights came on. Cynthia's relationship with her father was that of frequent confrontations, as he physically punished her for breaking house rules concerning curfew. According to Cynthia, physical punishment helped her to rationalize that it was better to remain away, having as much fun as possible. Thus, the corporal punishment's intent of forcing Cynthia to conform to conservative family norms actually drove her deeper into the streets.

> My daddy was real strict. Just didn't want me to be out there. My daddy didn't play nothing about us. I just wanted to be in the street. I wanted to hang with my friends and come in the house when I get ready. But they [her parents] weren't going for that. I had to be in the house before it get dark. I know I'm going to get a whipping so it make no sense in going [home]. I ain't fixin' to bring it to you. I already know I'm going to get a whipping so I just might as well stay on out. I say, "if they want me they'll come get me." You think I was fixin' to go home and know I'm fixin' to get a whipping? I stayed right on out there.

After receiving repeated whippings and punishments in terms of privileges being taking away, eventually Cynthia ran away. According to Cynthia, even as a middle-class teen, she fantasized about being a prostitute and living what she perceived to be a glamorous lifestyle. She recalled thinking about a woman she knew who prostituted herself and made three to four hundred dollars per trick. This woman that she looked up to on the streets used heroin and before long was injecting Cynthia. Cynthia said the pimps later learned that she was an underaged runaway and insisted that she return home before their operation was raided. While Cynthia went home for a few more years, she was still seeking to escape a controlling father, and decided to leave for Atlanta in 1979 to attend a vocational training program near the Rough. By the mid-1980s, she ended up in Atlanta, smoking crack cocaine and trying to maintain a relationship with a man whom she described as overbearing and violent at times.

Closely related to Cynthia's story, Peaches ran away from a rural-based middle-class home at the age of sixteen. However, Peaches was strategizing to escape sexual abuse at the hands of her stepfather. According to Peaches, her stepfather was an excellent economic provider as he was in the military and worked additional full-time jobs. Her mother owned a catering service and was often booked for years in advance for major events throughout their thriving middle-class community.

> He [my stepfather] was in the military. And he married my mama, and that's the only father I knew. . . . My life was good. My mama married a man that worked all the time just like she did. He was a good provider, but a Friday night drunk and Friday night fight every week. I didn't know whether to be happy or to be sad. Because we had whatever that people in our class could have. But every Friday night my daddy was going to get drunk at the Mug City before he came home. And then my father started drinking a lot and forgetting if I was my mother or if I was me. So all the good he did he erased in my heart or mind by getting drunk, coming in my room like he in the wrong room. But that June I left, because she loved him. She had to love him to stay with him when he beat her. Back then people stayed married regardless. You didn't hear about a lot of divorce or stuff like that. So they stayed together for forty-five years. So obvious to me he made her happy some kind of ways even though he made her sad. And she was determined that she was going to stick it out some way for us.

Peaches recalled how she came to realize that her mother would remain with her stepfather, primarily due to the economic stability he provided for the family. During this time, Peaches became promiscuous with older men outside the family and plotted to have one bring her to Atlanta and marry her. Peaches' story of sexual abuse at the hands of family members was echoed by several women in the Rough.

These women left home as early as fourteen years old to escape physical and sexual abuse; however, all of them ended up with older men who either abused them himself and or prostituted them. For these women, family relationships remain painful past memories as some family members fail to acknowledge in some cases, and minimize in other situations, the impact of the physical and sexual abuse these women endured as girls. Today, they are using crack cocaine to numb the pain when they really have unmet needs for treatment of post traumatic stress disorder.

Allison's upbringing mirrors Peaches' in that she also had a father who was an excellent economic provider, but terrorized the family with weekend fist fights with her mother. Allison describes her family life's frequent episodes of domestic violence.

> My mama moved to Atlanta. But my daddy wouldn't let us come. We knew that if we came up to Atlanta, daddy going to come up there and be still fighting. So we stayed with daddy. . . . My mama used to be so pretty. She went and got her hair fixed and all us children were standing and he took that water and throwed it in her face. My dad was so mean, he stunk. I caught him in the bed with a woman and he whipped me. My mama beat the brakes off him. My daddy was a rotten man. But my mama used to send us money from up here in Atlanta.

Allison went on to describe how her mother and father rotated between the city and the country over the years until Allison and her siblings finally settled in Atlanta with their father. By this time, as a single father, he raised them in a working-class neighborhood, where he worked a full-time job and ran a liquor house in the evenings and on the weekends. Allison assisted her father in selling liquor in the early 1980s, and when crack cocaine became available, she started selling this drug as well. Without the watchful eye of her mother, Allison remembers becoming more involved in the street life of the liquor house customers. While the other siblings were able to make a better transition into adulthood, Allison became further isolated from her family over the years.

> My daddy sold liquor and he worked. I was the worst mess in the world. But, other than that I got a good family. I love my

family. My family love me. If they can get me off drugs and get me [out the Rough]! They know something wrong with [me]. But they love me to death. And I look at myself sometimes and think about it. I got all this love. A lot of people ain't got no love, ain't got no home. They want me to come home.

Lolita's mother left her and her siblings with their grandparents when she was three years old. Throughout the community their family was known to be highly religious and hardworking. Lolita's childhood mental health was damaged as early as four years old when she vividly recalled her mother stating that she meant to have the first child, but that Lolita was a mistake. Mentally crippled by a mother's statements that she was an unwanted child, Lolita felt she had no one to turn to when her grandfather began molesting her in the basement. Lolita was confused about the sexual molestation because of the high-standing reputation her grandfather had in the family as a strong financial provider and preacher in the local church. Afraid of the unknown of where she would live if she revealed the sexual abuse, for years Lolita suffered in silence. She remembers how he approached her.

When I was five years old that man [her grandfather] ask me if I want to grow. I had them little school clothes with the strap come over the shoulder. Mine was too big. He asked me if I want to grow. He take me downstairs. They [the rest of the family] upstairs. They don't even know. Then when he took his thing out, he laid me on the bed. I grabbed him. Didn't nobody believe me but my uncle Malcolm. Man he whipped his ass somethin' else . . . And my grandma was so weak and she was so into the Lord she thought the Lord would handle it. When I turned twelve that's when he let me go back to my mama. By the time I turned twelve, I had it in my heart to kill his ass. 'Cause the next biscuit he ate was gonna be his damn last one. I had just that much hate in my heart. And then you get older and you still got to go through it.

Before Lolita could make good on her heart felt desire to kill her grandfather, her mother regained custody of her children, when Lolita was thirteen. However, by this time Lolita was mentally and emotionally scarred by repeated incidents of sexual abuse over a seven-year period, to the point that she was diagnosed as clinically depressed and mildly retarded later in life and even spent time in a mental institution.

Gloria's father was a pastor of a church who remained in touch with her after her parents divorced. She recalls spending time with him on the weekends, but did not feel any emotional attachment to him or his new family. She became very tearful in describing how hurt she was when her father didn't express his feelings toward her when she became pregnant as a teen.

> Me and my father love each other, but we're just not like a father and daughter. I'm the oldest, so it's not like that bond that a father usually has with a daughter. When I got pregnant the first time to me it seem like it didn't matter either way it went, whether I was pregnant or not.

Gloria appears to believe that there is a "typical" father-daughter relationship which she perceives as not having developed between her and her father. Perhaps she felt the most disappointment when her father showed no reactions to becoming a grandfather. Gloria's narrative suggests that she would have appreciated any kind of reaction—positive or negative. This desperate need for attention is common among girls suffering from severe abandonment. For his part, perhaps because of his profession as a pastor, Gloria's father tried to downplay the fact that his daughter had broken one of the Christian and middle-class taboos against teen pregnancy. In any case, Gloria continues to have unmet needs related to her feelings that her father abandoned her.

Teresa, now a 36-year-old mother of five, actually grew up middle class in the Rough during the late seventies and early eighties, at a time when there still was a thriving and visible black middle class in the area. She was bussed to a predominantly white high school and her parents are well-known and respected business owners in the community. Teresa was very defensive about the neighborhood, as she was socialized around others in the Rough who were middle-class African Americans. She succumbed to a life of daily drug use after losing what she described as a good job at the bank.

People over here not poor. They might live in a poor neighborhood, but believe me, they a long way from being poor. They
living better than millionaires over here. I done went through
some houses where you think they was poor and these were millionaires. They living in a old dirty ran-down house.

Teresa's comments at best represent an exaggerated recollection of
her middle class upbringing in the Rough. At worst she has grossly
failed to observe the Rough's shift from a community where middle
class families once lived to one where poverty is severe and highly
concentrated. In either case, I spent time dialoguing with Teresa on
my thoughts about the community as a poor neighborhood. She defended her perception of the Rough as a neighborhood where people
"look poor," but actually have "millions of dollars." In a very frustrated tone, I "schooled" Teresa on the realities of the Rough as a poor
community:

This would be classified as a poor neighborhood when you speak
of it in relations to a middle class neighborhood or an upper class
neighborhood. And by all the measures of poverty, [the Rough]
is considered poor. We measure poverty by income and the up
keep of the neighborhood. And quite frankly it's not just the
people around here who are responsible for this being labeled as
a poverty neighborhood. If you take jobs away and send them
overseas people are gonna be unemployed. If you take away the
incentive for the people to keep up their taxes in the neighborhood they are not going to pay them because they don't see the
city investing in the schools. So then people move out and they
let people rent their houses and they don't come back and fix
them up.

Despite my attempt to provide a definition and even suggest that
the Rough became a poor neighborhood over time because of government decisions to move jobs and training programs out of reach, Teresa
remained defensive about my statements of the Rough as a poor community. Teresa was the only woman who perceived the Rough to be
anything other than mired in poverty. So, for the most part, the realities of the Rough as a community of joblessness, drug-infestation,

and shrinking property values are clearly observable by the other women.

Women from decent families for the most part provided stories that left their parents blameless in their own choices to use drugs and have unsafe sex. For example, Pauline, a 32-year-old mother of two, remained in the Rough with her father after her parents divorced. She described herself as a "good girl" with a "good background," which includes two years of college education. In fact, six other women had at least two years of college education. Like Pauline, these women perceive themselves to have been successfully socialized as products of decent families in the Rough. Pauline admits to having tried drugs after completing high school and starting her first year of college. Her drug of choice was cocaine stuffed in a cigarette or marijuana, often referred to as a "geek joint." She stopped using drugs for three years while she worked and attended college. Pauline recalls her relapse.

> [I] stayed right in the Rough all my life and [my father] was my everything. He never hit me. I used to be a good girl. I had a good background. Graduated [from high school]. I went to college for two years. When I was eighteen I was off and on [drugs]. And I stopped three years on my own. Then I had a relapse. I was working at the hotel and going to school at nighttime. I switched up going to school in the day. And one night I spent my whole check. I had a relapse. The next morning I was getting ready to go to work. I felt like nothing. I kept working and then I stopped.

After Pauline stopped working and going to school, she started hustling drugs with her brother. According to Pauline, "I was the youngest one up there on that corner. I was making $10,000 a week. I had five cars and a townhouse." From there she remembers being in and out of jail for drug charges, and eventually began using more drugs than she was selling. At one point, she owed so much money for drugs on credit she could not be seen on the streets she once dominated as a drug dealer in the Rough.

Dee-Dee, a 50-year-old mother of two adult daughters who are married and living in Texas, is originally from a rural county in Georgia. She came to Atlanta on a sports scholarship and later dropped out of college. She managed to go to trade school as an interior decorator and master chef. She ended up in the Rough five years ago, but had been coming to the neighborhood to buy drugs for years. Having raised her own children in the suburbs, she attempts to provide a sense of community for the children in the neighborhood. Dee-Dee believes that many of their parents are using drugs and attempts to make her house a safe place to play after school.

> I've been living over here about five years but I've been coming over here forever. And all the kids in the neighborhood know me and when they get out of school, imagine fifty-eight children coming to your house every day 'cause I got to have them cake or whatever. I do birthday parties for 'em, put on my clown out-fit. I get out there and turn flips with them. I take 'em to the parks. Stuff that I did with my kids and these kids don't get a chance to do it.

Johnsie, a 37-year-old mother of four, grew up in rural Georgia. She left home to escape being molested by her birth father. After moving to Florida, she married a man and later served seven years in jail for attempting to murder him and a woman she caught him with in her house. Upon being released from jail at age twenty-eight she came to the Rough, where her mother was living at the time. She began selling drugs with her brother and eventually was using more crack than she was selling. Her mother has since relocated Johnsie's children to a suburb of Atlanta; however, Johnsie remains on the streets of the Rough.

Doll, originally from the suburbs of Chicago, first came to a suburb of Georgia after completing high school to attend college and live with her mother and grandmother. Doll ended up in the Rough one year ago after leaving her boyfriend, who introduced her to drug selling and using. Unlike the typical street corner drug dealer, Doll's boyfriend set up legitimate businesses, and given her business degree, she was able to serve as a manager and bookkeeper. In the early years she was sheltered from the drug distribution aspects and was able to present an image of successful business owner to her mainstream family and friends until she began using drugs.

Women who defined their families of orientation as decent tended to stress the importance of economic stability as a key characteristic that separated them from street families. However, the extent of sexual and physical abuse reported separately by these women cannot be ignored as a key factor that must be addressed in taking steps toward building these women's self-worth, which would ultimately result in enhanced empowerment to take back ownership of their bodies. Their narratives suggest that black girls raised in families labelled decent from an economic standpoint, remain at high risk for sexual molestation in ways that may manifest later as part and parcel of one's engaging in high-risk behavior. These women's socialization as black girls in decent families highlights key areas of vulnerability.

GROWING UP STREET

There were sixteen women who described themselves as having grown up "street," hustling, pimping, and drugs being part of their families' daily lives. As some women are products of two generations of welfare dependency, they know only chronic economic and social instability as part of their upbringing. As children, these women remember lives of high levels of economic and social instability, and they speak of having to be resilient and resourceful at an early age in order to survive. Many of these women tended to change residency frequently as children, with each move being brought on by the reescalation of violence or limited financial resources. Because of the change of address, many changed schools as much as three times in one school year. Furthermore, women who grew up street highlighted long periods of parental neglect, with some spending most of their formative years in foster care. As children, many women who grew up street witnessed having one or both parents serve jail time. Still, others were personally affected by the AIDS virus in the early 1980s, as they have parents who were IDUs (intravenous drug users). Others grew up in homes where drug selling and using, as well as child prostitution, was thrust on them at very early ages by their own parents. Still other street women recall becoming teen mothers as early as thirteen years old.

Writing the stories of women who grew up street brought on a level of anxiety I had not expected. From a cultural standpoint, I was paralyzed by the unwritten rule among African Americans that no matter the degree or detriment, we don't air our dirty laundry for all to read and critique. Politically, I wanted to guard against giving either the morally or fiscally conservative even the smallest amount of information that could be used to support their arguments of criminalization of these women's behavior as part of a pathological upbringing. However, as a black feminist, I felt compelled to give full and honest accounts of women who grew up street. In the end, I concluded that it is better to speak the truth about this group of women's high-risk childhoods in a way that provides an insider's perspective into how girls become entangled in the "family businesses" of drug selling and prostitution. So, at the risk of being criticized as politically incorrect or culturally insensitive, I chose to give voice to the stories many wish would not be told. My motive for telling their stories is to inform the next generation of HIV prevention interventions that focus on building HIV prevention capacity in communities where risky behavior is normalized in key socializing institutions. In the end, we cannot reclaim what we will not name. If we want to reclaim our inner cities, then we must stop being ashamed of the women's realities in the streets.

Women described how growing up street sometimes resulted in parents introducing their children to drug selling and drug using. In this way, these girls were deprived of their own opportunities to have childhood dreams about what they wanted to be when they grew up, as their first jobs in the illegal drug economy would shape their future forever. For example, Erica grew up in the heart of the Rough and was socialized around the inner workings of her father's heroin and crack cocaine business. She dropped out of high school in the mid-1980s, and had been selling marijuana since middle school when she stole her mother's drugs. Later, her father recruited four of his six children into the drug-dealing business. According to Erica, all four of them later became drug users.

> We were born in this [drug dealing business]. My daddy was a major heroin dealer in Atlanta. And I was the first one who got off into the [drug dealing business]. I started selling heroin when I dropped out of school. He told me I couldn't stay at home and spend him and mama money and not work. I tried to work at a McDonald's and I didn't like that. So I started to bag [put drugs in individual small containers for distribution] and that was for my allowance. [I] was getting like two hundred bucks a week and at sixteen that was major money. Then not to mention I was

cheating him out of his [drugs] too. Daddy was illiterate. I'm
stashing bags and shit and everything. And that's how I got
started. We was making major money over there. We was selling
crack. We was making like fifteen thou[sand] a day. Me and my
mom and my brother. I mean we done that [sold drugs] faith-
fully for like nine years.

At the height of the "New Jack" era in the mid-1980s, Erica recalls
almost every corner in the Rough being occupied day and night by
young children operating in different roles as part of the family business of drug dealing. She recalls how boys as young as ten were recruited by their own family members to be lookouts and to run drugs
and money in backpacks. While young boys had dreams of getting rich
quick, as evident in making one hundred dollars per day for merely
watching and running, most girls in this environment had ambitions
to be the leading lady of a big time drug dealer, and many were encouraged by their mothers to date only "men with money." Some
girls, however, such as Erica, were just as hard as the boys and
wanted to make their own money in the drug business. Erica and her
family were selling drugs out of a government project in the Rough
and were later evicted under harsh public housing covenants against
the selling of drugs on the premises. According to Erica, she became
sloppy in handling the drug business, as she began smoking as much
crack as she sold. She recalls being so careless that she would be
smoking crack outside knowing she had "thousands of dollars" in
crack inside the house. She demonstrated how she was taking her last
hit as a free woman even when the police were kicking the door down
with a search warrant. As a result, Erica served three years in the peni-
tentiary and returned to her grandmother's house in the Rough where
her sister and mother had been since getting evicted earlier.

Erica's mother, Mattie, also grew up in the Rough and was a participant in the HIP project. However, Mattie adamantly denies selling
crack cocaine with Erica and her brother. According to Mattie, she
had lived in the same housing project for thirty-two years and worked
as a hairdresser. In the late 1970s she admits cooking and packaging
heroin for her husband. She also sold marijuana, which she says Erica
began stealing and selling at school at age thirteen. Mattie's account
of Erica's upbringing was one of trying to make a "lady" out of her,
but that Erica insisted on being a drug dealer. Making a lady out of her

meant preparing her to be a leading lady by knowing how to account for drug sells, serving as the front person for business investments with drug money, and providing a happy home for drug dealers. In preparation for Erica to become a leading lady, Mattie bought her two girls the latest fashions, musical instruments, and characterized herself as a hands-on parent who was very involved in her children's education. She believes she provided a good home for her three children and is perplexed as to why the girls made what she considers bad choices. On the other hand, her son lives in a middle-class neighborhood and earns a living wage as a blue-collar worker. According to Mattie, her children had more than most growing up in the Rough during the eighties. She believes this may have spoiled them, and hindered their willingness to work a wage-paying job, as they were accustomed to material things being given to them from "fast money."

Janice was raised in the streets by a mother who drank alcohol and lived with an abusive partner. Janice's biological father attempted to rescue his children from this environment, but was only able to temporarily shelter them at his sister's house. Eventually, Janice and her siblings returned to live with their abusive stepfather and mother.

> My mom raised us, but I had a stepdad, but he was really a woman beater. He used to beat my mom all the time. And we were too young to do anything about it. That went on for some years 'til we got like thirteen or fourteen years old, 'til we moved with my dad. Me, my sister and brother—we moved with my daddy in Eastlake Meadows. That was really my aunt house, but he was staying with her, but anyway my stepdad broke my mom arm, broke one of her arms and one of her legs and her jaw. So after that incident happen they came and got all of us, you know. Wasn't no kids born then [her children]. I think my sister was pregnant with her first one then, you know. But anyway my dad came and got me, my sister, brother, and my mom. And my mom when she got well, she went right back over there. Yeah, that's normal, 'cause she love him, that's who she want to be with. And he talked her down, and said he wouldn't go do it no more.

As Janice's narrative indicates, she now reflects on the violent encounters between her mother and stepfather as "normal." Having been

socialized to believe that domestic violence is normal in relationships, Janice herself has maintained a five-year relationship with a
male batterer. Her biological father eventually moved Janice in with
his sister, but this change of residency only served to expose Janice to
another aspect of street life, as her father sold drugs, and over time
Janice began selling crack with her father and brother. According to
Janice, she started selling marijuana first. Then she saw her other family members making much more money selling crack. She remembers it being the norm to give the babysitter crack cocaine as payment
for her babysitting services. She moved from being a drug seller to
user as her stepmother offered her crack cocaine to ease the pain of a
headache.

> I had just had my first son and she used to do the Coca Cola
> cans. And I used to have these young dope boys and stuff. I used
> to come in the house 'cause I might have some dope and stuff
> and I used to give it to them. I say, you want this, what you want.
> Or I may give it to the babysitter or something. But back then
> I didn't know they were dime sacks. I was giving up like four or
> five sacks, giving up dope like that. But one time I gave her like
> five sacks, five dimes and left with the girls. For some reason
> I just didn't feel good or something. She say you want these
> bags?

As Janice explains, drugs among street families serve several pur-
poses. On the one hand, they do provide a steady cash flow. However,
they can be used to barter needed services, such as babysitting in this
case. In addition, there were several women who discussed using
crack cocaine as a form of self-medication.

To be fair, adolescents across race and class lines report using drugs
as part of their typical social setting. However, there is no denying that
for street children, drug using among peers can be more detrimental.
Shanté was socialized in a home where drug using among friends and
relatives was the norm. In such an environment, Shanté began smoking marijuana as early as middle school and began selling it in high
school for her mother and older brothers. Shanté recalled how her
brother and his friends accused her of being antisocial because she
smoked her marijuana in a separate room from them. According to

Shanté, she knew they were smoking crack cocaine and was trying to avoid this drug as she already knew how addictive crack cocaine was by observing her customers. Over time, however, Shanté gave into the peer pressure.

> I used to just sit upstairs and smoke reefa [marijuana]. One day my brother [and his friends] was all over our house. I used to sell the reefa and I had my li'l plain joint. They was in the other room. They talkin' 'bout, "you being antisocial." I'm steady tryin' to look and make sure they don't pass me the wrong joint. Somebody caught my attention and they passed me the wrong joint. Ever since then [I been smoking crack].

Tomeka remembers her childhood in the Rough and being introduced to drugs, alcohol, and prostitution as a normal part of growing up in the streets. Tomeka's own mother was a prostitute and alcoholic. Tomeka attributes her first experiments with drugs to an attempt to mask the pain associated with her relationship with her mother. She recalls how her mother would use her as a child to service customers who preferred sex with a young girl.

> She got angry with me because she taught me how to prostitute in my younger days. But if the dude didn't have no sex with me she used to get the guys to take me up to somebody's house. Then take me and put me under the bed and get the man's money out of the pocket.

Tomeka eventually became pregnant and gave birth to her only child at age sixteen. She started smoking crack cocaine at twenty-four and took her first hit of heroin four years later when her sister and cousin convinced her to allow them to shoot her up. As she reflects on the Rough some thirty years after growing up there, she believes that bad parenting resulted in her high-risk behavior. Tomeka's point of view is that the neighborhood is a reflection of the people who live there. As she considers herself to be a victim of bad parenting, she believes that high-risk drug and sexual behavior is learned from parents. However, Tomeka's account of the Rough as a bad neighborhood because of poor parenting is unique in that no other woman blamed her parents for her own high-risk behavior.

Punkin described herself as being the daughter of a street woman and living off and on with relatives who often prophesized that she would follow in her mother's footsteps. Punkin was able to temporarily escape life on the streets with her mother when she opted to move in with her father and stepmother. Early on Punkin recognized a difference in the treatment she received from her stepmother in comparison to the way that her stepmother treated her own biological children. This led to Punkin running away to escape the physical and emotional pain of living in a home where she observed other children being nurtured and loved, but not feeling the same acceptance herself.

> I didn't agree with the setting at home, and moved away [from] my stepmother and her children. I didn't agree with how she treated me. And I was abused as a child. And she didn't do nothing, 'cause I was not her child. But I had a choice. I wanted to be with my father. But if I knew it was goin' to be like this, I would never even be talking to you.

MAKING SENSE OF DECENT AND STREET UPBRINGING

Collectively, the women in this study confirm that for black girls, there are blurred lines between decent and street family life. Their stories challenge us to look beyond economic stability as a single indicator for child well-being, and begin to examine the interconnectedness of economic stability, emotional support, and exposure to sexual exploitation and domestic violence as multiple indicators of future risk and protection against HIV among black girls. Clearly, a glimpse into these women's accounts of their childhood private lives inside middle-class families suggest that economic stability serves as a buffer between middle-class black families and child protection services in ways that actually may increase prolonged and escalated experiences of child sexual abuse in the privacy of decent family homes. Many women from decent upbringings revealed family secrets in their lives as girls as they struggle to make sense of a family environment that was economically secure, yet sexually unsafe.

In comparison, the street women discussed drug use and drug selling as being a normal part of their socialization process. Several women could only idealize a life with mainstream middle-class constructs where parents worked living wage jobs, did not sell or use drugs, and valued educational attainment if not for themselves, at least for their children. No matter whether these women are from decent or street families, there is a need to provide a space in HIV prevention for them to discuss the ways in which they were socialized to give meaning to drug using, drug selling and sexual activities. This information provides insight for more effective individualized plans for HIV prevention.

In examining these women's narratives, I discovered women who had never had an opportunity to process the idea that past family secrets are interconnected to their current risk for HIV. Their voices and feelings concerning being sexually abused have been silenced first in their homes and later in their adult lives. The prevalence of sexual abuse is evident in both decent and street families. In general, however, child sexual abuse is underreported, and even more so in middle class families where economic stability often provides a privilege of privacy where family secrets are more likely to be shielded. Despite this prevalence, researchers have only recently begun to focus on the long-term consequences of child sexual abuse (Kelly, 2003; Ladwig and Andersen, 1989). The majority of research suggests that a variety of negative psychological, behavioral, and interpersonal problems are more prevalent among incest victims than among individuals without such a history. The long-term effects on sexually abused children include a large percentage becoming prostitutes and drug users, activities that place them at higher risk for HIV (Kelly, 2003; Ladwig and Andersen, 1989).

ACCOUNTS OF INTERACTIONS WITH FAMILIES OF ORIENTATION

In this section, women provide accounts of current interactions with their families of orientation. The analysis for these narratives centers on examining specific strengths and barriers in women's familial relationships that may impact the women's motivation for setting and achieving HIV prevention goals and strategies. There were four dominant themes used to describe women's attachment and interaction with their families: (1) missing significant deceased family members, (2) avoiding interaction with family, (3) deceiving family, and (4) engaging in frequent interaction with family.

Missing Significant Deceased Family

Losing significant family members to death has an impact on women's risky behavior. The family members women missed the most were their mothers, sisters, and fathers. These family members in particular are characterized as supporting women financially and emotionally and may have cared for the women's minor children. Not coping adequately with the death of a family member leads to increases in high-risk behavior among women already doing drugs or engaging in high-risk sex. Pauline is one such woman, raised by her father, who felt she was unable to really focus on doing anything positive for herself because she was still processing the loss of her father. She is still trying to gain the mental strength to deal with his death.

> My daddy died three years ago now. He was my everything; my best friend. Never denied me for nothing. He never hit me for nothing. He never demanded me. Just had me spoiled. And without him I can't seem to regain the strength back. And I'm going through a whole lot.

Doll had a similarly strong relationship with her mother and grandmother, and after their deaths, Doll became more integrated into the drug-using network for emotional support. She remembers trying to talk to one of the risk reduction counselors as a substitute for discussing issues she had previously discussed with her mother and grandmother.

> I'm mainly missing my mama and my grandmama. They say when your mama gone you ain't got nobody and that's the truth. There's nobody I can really go and see about [her problems]. I could come and talk to [one of the counselors], but it's still not like talking with my grandma; talk with my mama. It still some things you scared to even say to somebody. I'm trying to get back to where I was.

Mona was raised in the foster care system in New York, where she was separated from her blood sister for over eight years. After she turned eighteen, Mona came to Atlanta to be with her baby sister, who was the only biological family member she remained in touch with while in foster care. Mona remembers her sister being involved in a relationship that was intensely violent; ultimately her sister died of a brain aneurysm. Mona admits that she and her sister were drinking and smoking together, but she maintained a job in security at the airport. After her sister died, Mona's life spiraled out of control and she ended up homeless under a bridge.

Women who discussed the death of their family members talked about feeling guilty for not attending family funerals and for not fulfilling promises made to close relatives to stop using drugs. For these high-risk women, close deceased family members represent the only person these women believe cared for them. So, when these particular family members die, the women discussed increased high-risk behavior for extended periods as a way to mask the pain and cope with loss.

Wanda was the only person who described using her mother's death as inspiration in a sense to decrease her risky behavior. Wanda started to make changes after she made a promise to her mother that she would stop using drugs. Wanda explains, "I wish I still had a mama. She been dead nine years . . . and I had promised her I was going to slow down when she was alive . . . It don't even phase me no more."

Several women who cared for sick and aging family members that ultimately died reject the discourse that long-time crack users fail to function as caregivers within the family unit. In general, drug addiction literature often characterizes crack-using women as selfish and incapable of effectively managing daily routines and responsibilities. Several of the women described specific examples of how they nurtured family members through sickness and old age and even handled the details related to the funeral services. Stephanie talked about her caregiving experiences for her HIV-positive siblings:

> I took care of my brother and my sister. I took care of them until they died. I changed their diapers and fed them. That's why when anybody say anything negative about people with AIDS I'm ready to knock a stick over their head.

Pamela is another example of a woman who balanced the roles of family caregiver and drug user. Not only did Pamela tend to her ailing mother, but after her mother died, she moved her 72-year-old father to Atlanta from Iowa.

> My mama got sick and I knew she had cancer, but I didn't know it was in the advanced stages. So when she called me, she said, I'm fine baby girl. I said, mama I think I need to come home. She died in May . . . My mom passed. I took a drug overdose so that knocked me off the box then . . . I think [my father] grieved himself to death. I got him and brought him down here. That's before they foreclosed on my house. He got down here and he had a stroke . . . We cut the plug off on him last Tuesday and . . . buried him Friday. I'm here and I'm smiling 'cause I know they in a better place and not suffering.

Caring for her mom who was HIV positive resulted in Sonya lowering her own risky behavior, as the time she normally spent in the streets was now directed toward taking care of her mom. According to Sonya, she was unable to truly focus on getting high because she needed to be alert in tending to her mother's medical needs. When I spoke with her for this project, Sonya's mother was in the hospital in intensive care. Sonya had been sleeping at the hospital for the last two weeks as her mother drifted in and out of consciousness. Sonya explained that she has known for sometime that both of her parents were HIV positive, and she was prepared for their deaths.

Shanté remembers how part of her everyday life growing up revolved around canvassing the neighborhood looking for her mother at various shooting galleries. One of the worst nights, however, was having to pull her mother out of the bushes after the people in the shooting gallery pushed her outside in her wheelchair for fear that she would die of an overdose in the house.

> I done seen where she done OD'd [overdosed]. They had to bring her back. They left her for dead one time . . . I had found her. Something had done told me to walk 'round the building and it was dark. I heard something moaning in the corner. It was like by some bushes. And she was in a wheelchair. There was my mama and I had to get her and bring her back. She had done

went out [nodded out] in somebody house and they was scared. They put her in the wheelchair and pushed her out the door.

According to Shanté, these types of encounters became the norm for coping with her mother's heroin addiction. Her mother later became HIV positive and as the disease progressed, she was hospitalized and eventually died of heart failure. Shanté spent the next few days collecting donations from individuals in the neighborhood to bury her mother.

> She didn't have no insurance. I had to raise three thousand dollars to bury my mama. I got it. I guess God was with me. It took two or three days but I did it.

Karen's mother has been deceased for nine years, and her father is in a home for the disabled, as he is blind. Karen's baby sister recently moved in with her, and now that she has AIDS, she needs more assistance in her everyday life. Karen remembers how before her sister moved in with her, she was sleeping on the street and in abandoned apartments after losing her own government-sponsored housing.

> I told my sister you ain't gotta live like this, but it took me a while to get her from off in there. I had got tired. I left her alone. One day I came home from the club, she was sitting' there on my steps.

These women's strengths as nurturers and caregivers to adult family members often is overlooked as a motivation for setting HIV risk reduction goals. As these women articulated, they found a sense of value and self-worth in caring for family members. When these ailing or aged family members die, however, these women lose the status of caregiver, which changes their daily routine, as they no longer have to ensure that these family members eat or bathe, or accompany them to doctor's visits and assure they take their medication regularly.

Avoiding Interaction with Family

Many of the women described how they avoid interaction with their family because they are ashamed of themselves as drug-using

women and mothers in particular. Pauline expressed being ashamed
of her personal appearance. When I asked Pauline about her mother,
she teared up and expressed, "It's been so long, it's ugly. She love me,
I just can't face her. I'm ashamed." Martha provided a similar story of
being ashamed.

> I got two brothers and I got two sisters here [in Georgia] and
> I got one sister in Houston. They might be worried about me
> and I just don't want them to see me right now. I don't look like
> I used to before I got on drugs. I don't dress like I use to. I'm just
> a different person. I always dressed neat. My hair always stayed
> neat. I had beautiful black skin. Everything just done changed.
> And I always had a good job, a nice home. So right now, I just
> don't want them to see me.

Even though Dorothy is in the process of recovering from drugs
and has improved her personal appearance, she continues to avoid
contact with her family. She expressed a desire to reunite with her
family in Iowa, where her four children are now twenty-one, twenty-
two, twenty-four, and twenty-six. She has not contacted them in ten
years, but believes that now she has cleaned up and can face them.
Dorothy recognizes that they may not welcome her with open arms,
and she wants to be prepared for that. She understands that such rejection from loved ones could trigger a relapse due to feelings of
unworthiness. Therefore, she wants to wait until she has "enough recovery in me so I can tell them what I went through."

Tracie has attempted to be drug free and even left Baltimore to
come to Atlanta, believing that a change of environment would help
her to maintain her commitment to be drug free. She is embarrassed
that she is the only one in her family on drugs and continues to avoid
contact with her family until she is cleaned up.

> I'm the youngest of five. Out of the five I'm the only one that
> uses drugs . . . I have a beautiful relationship with my family.
> My family wants me to come home. That's what they want me
> to do but I don't want to go home because I refuse to go home
> the way that I left. I took them through hell. Thank God for a
> forgivin' family. They still love me. They want me to come home
> and get myself together.

Even though some women avoid their family members because they are ashamed, these women hold onto beliefs that their family loves them and wants to see them clean. Like Tracie, Lisa is the only one in her family who smokes crack. Unlike Tracie, however, Lisa believes her family is totally unaware of her crack habit. While Lisa doesn't avoid her family physically as the other women in this category do, she does avoid disclosing the fact that she smokes crack cocaine. She explains why it is important that she hides her crack use from her family.

> The only thing they know is like we all, drink. All my sisters and brothers 'drink. None of them know about me smoking [crack]. And boy I'll probably have to lay down in a grave if they do know because they those type of people. My family where I grew up, that's unacceptable. I'll be sitting in my mama house, all of us be sitting around and somebody come on TV and the first they say is, oh she must be on dope and then they go talking about it real bad. I sit right there. And one time I heard my mama say, Oh I had this friend and I found out she was on dope and I cut her loose—ain't nothing I can do for them people like that. Only thing I can do is call somebody for you, but me, I can't deal with you. But guess what? You got a daughter. What if I told her I was on dope? What, you going to just push me off too and tell me, I can't deal with you. I sit there and I listen to them talk and I sit there. I mean its kind of depressing in a way then I sit there hearing them saying that. If they aren't going to help and if I did want to get off, if I did want to get my life together I couldn't go to them.

DECEIVING FAMILY MEMBERS

Deceiving concerned mothers who would do anything to help their daughters has served as a major source of conflict between high-risk women and their families of orientation. Over time, however, these women's mothers grow tired of the lies and deceit and eventually stop believing in their daughters' ability to make positive changes in their lives. Having no family support after mothers end communication and contact, these women face heightened risk for HIV infection because they no longer have access to a safe place to take a break from drugs and turning dates, or to get food and a shower. At this point, these women must increase their dependence on street-based networks for their daily living as well as for the kind of emotional support often provided by one's family of orientation. Portia describes how she took advantage of her mother's willingness to assist her financially.

> I done told her every lie in the book . . . I can get her to send me a hundred dollars, two hundred, but it's not worth it. When she don't send me [money] I get mad and won't call her. So she hurries up and sends it.

Johnsie echoed Portia's story of how high-risk women deceive their mothers in particular with elaborate schemes concerning money.

> One time me and Mama had a argument. She had gave me some money for myself. I begged her for it. I told her, when I come back it's going to be more. I can pay her back. And it was one of her bill money and she trusted me. She gave it to me and instead of me doing what I told her I was gonna do I smoked it. So she came and when she came I didn't have [the money]. She say, git your ass in this car. My Mama took me out in the woods and I thought, Mama fixin' to kill me. My Mama cussed my out for days. She made me feel this little.

ENGAGING IN FREQUENT INTERACTION WITH FAMILY

Several women in the Rough maintain relations with their families of orientation. Some of these women provided accounts of very positive interactions with their family members in ways that could serve as sources of strength and inspiration for those committed to reducing their high-risk behavior. Their stories provide a perspective that even as chronic crack users, these women are able to express feelings of love, respect, commitment, and responsibility to other family members, albeit on a limited basis. Nevertheless, such positive interaction gives the HIV prevention planner additional opportunities to enhance individual HIV prevention goals and objectives among women who have positive relations with their families of orientation. For example, Shanese was excited to let me know that she had a 1:30 p.m. engagement to participate in a family dinner for her mother. Shanese remains in the Rough because she is determined to try and make her intimate relationship work, but maintains contact with her family. She even alluded to the fact that she is tired of the continued turmoil with her intimate partner and may rely on the close relationship she has with her mother as a way out.

Jennifer discussed how her self-worth was enhanced by increasing the time she spent with her family of orientation. According to Jennifer, she felt like her family did not love her any longer after learning of her drug use. However, in the last year, her family started to provide emotional support and she increased the time she spent around them. This meant that Jennifer had less time on the streets, and in her own words, "I ain't out on the street as much. I started back caring 'bout myself. . . . My family love me when I start loving myself."

Daisy returned home to live with her mother after losing a living wage job in 1990. Daisy rationalized that since her mother was aging, and the neighborhood was growing more dangerous, it was better that she move home to take care of her mother. However, Daisy admits that being at home with no financial resources of her own has brought on more stress. As her other family members do not use drugs or smoke cigarettes, she has to take to the streets to interact with a network of individuals who can supply these habits. From Daisy's perspective, she believes that because she cares for her mother, she should be allowed to eat whatever is available in the kitchen. According to Daisy, when her mother and other family members complain that she is eating too much food without contributing financially, she is inclined to leave the house and take to the streets in ways that heighten her risk for HIV infection.

This chapter confirms the need for more in-depth research into the private lives of middle-class black families as a way of explaining why financial stability as a predictor of positive child outcomes needs to be contextualized, particularly in the lives of black girls, who are at higher risk for sexual abuse in their homes than are black boys. These women's comments about their families of orientation help us to understand how families shape the environment and everyday lives of women's current risk behaviors, as well as their degrees of motivation to change. For example, keeping secrets in middle-class black families concerning child sexual abuse in the lives of girls results in abused adolescents who arrive at adulthood not having properly processed the abused self. Many of these girls begin acting out on their abused self in ways that are labeled promiscuous, with many leaving the familial environments that proved limited in providing the safety and security that is idealized as the norm in our society. Just like their street cohorts, many girls from decent families who face child sexual abuse succumb to substance abuse, depression, and feelings of helplessness that manifest in low educational attainment, limited employment choices, and bad intimate relationships.

There were three main standpoints that became clear for me after analyzing these women's historical accounts of growing up and ending up in the Rough. First, I believe those who grew up in the Rough and Rough-like communities are more likely to believe that they can make changes and maintain in the Rough. At first I felt their statements such as "the neighborhood is alright," and "it's millionaires live over here" were made in defense of my direct and indirect accusations that the Rough is a high-risk, poverty-stricken community. However, a closer examination of these women's comments suggests that they sincerely believe themselves to be strong enough to make positive changes within this socially constructed "bad neighborhood."

The second standpoint is centered on the unique characteristics among seemingly heterogeneous groups. For example, I had begun my inquiry with the notion that these were all poor, underprivileged women with limited opportunities for higher education and who were victims of seemingly insurmountable structural constraints. By the end, however, I understood the value of black feminism as it relates to self-definition and self-valuation in the lives of African-American women. While they were all poor African-American women who use crack when I met them in the Rough, they often defined themselves as "who they once were" in comparison to "who they have become." Thus, a black feminist perspective helped me to approach my study with more respect and patience in allowing the women to construct an image of themselves that differed from my initial tendency to assume they all grew up poor and at risk in the Rough or Rough-like areas. In addition, I learned that to approach these women as if they were reared in poverty, when in fact they were not, can be insulting and may result in losing their trust and respect.

The third standpoint is that helping the women think through their experiences as children and adolescents and how they arrived at their present state can be extremely helpful in getting them to think about and subsequently change behaviors that they conclude are harmful to themselves (Fullilove et al., 1993; Fullilove, Lown, and Fullilove, 1992; Fagan and Chin, 1989). For example, in the early months of working in the HIP House, it was obvious that I was outraged at the stronghold of drugs in the community in general and in the lives of these women in particular. However, I had to learn to respect that whether they were socialized in the Rough as adults or as children, it was their life and their story. In like manner, it was their choice to change. While I could be a facilitator of thought and change, the actual new thoughts and changed actions had to be initiated and implemented by the women themselves. Once I toned down my own outrage and sense of hopelessness as I interacted with the women, I noticed that I was invited further into the HIP House experience. Both the staff and the women saw me as someone who respected where the women were in their lives, as well as how they had gotten there.

PRINCIPLES TO GUIDE FAMILY-FOCUSED HIV PREVENTION INITIATIVES

It is clear that women in this study would benefit from at least one family member of orientation understanding the process associated with HIV prevention among crack-using women. As high-risk behavior and activities are normalized among acquaintances in the drug-using networks, these women are in need of positive social networks to replace those they come to rely on in high-risk settings. Members of one's family of orientation can serve as a substitute for one's current reliance on members of high-risk social networks. I call this "social replacement theory," in that individuals need a person or group of people to fill the social void left in one's daily life when they disengage from their high-risk social network as part of risk reduction. At the same time, family members who serve in a social replacement capacity need to be aware of what the high-risk woman may be experiencing and how they can serve as a change agent that helps bridge the gap of social isolation as women transition out of high-risk social networks. Family members can also serve as mediators between the high-risk woman and other family members who may need to be involved in the HIV prevention process.

Family-focused interventions in HIV prevention typically have centered on strategies to help individuals in the gay community come out to their families in hopes that such an event will result in lowered risk behavior (Kadushin, 1996). Others have been counseled as part of their HIV prevention case management on how to cope with continued rejection from one's family of orientation in ways that do not place them at heightened risks for HIV infection (Kadushin, 1996). Unlike the gay community, however, black women's family relationships often are further complicated because various family members may be caring for the women's minor children (Dancy, Marcantonio, and Norr, 2000). However, black women are not counseled on how to cope with rejection and ridicule by family members as part of their HIV prevention.

HIV prevention programs must help high-risk women process how losing significant family members can increase their risk for HIV infection if they cope with loss by increasing their high-risk behavior. Men in general are not typically socialized to take on the responsibility of caring for the sick and aging in their family. Acting as caregivers for aging extended family members is often a unique experience among African-American women, so there is a need for HIV prevention programs to address diverse family relationships that may be serving as barriers and facilitators for HIV risk behaviors.

As HIV and drug abuse continue to cripple the black family in general, in ways that threaten future generations, there needs to be a greater sense of urgency among HIV prevention researchers to plan and implement family-focused HIV prevention interventions that are cost-effective for families with limited resources. These women's narratives suggest that family relationships can serve as barriers and facilitators of HIV prevention. For example, women who describe positive relationships with their family of orientation should be encouraged to incorporate their family members into their HIV risk reduction plans. At the same time, women who view family encounters as more stressful experiences should be counseled on how such interactions may result in high-risk behavior as they attempt to de-stress themselves.

The core theme is that there are differences in family relations among these women and thus HIV prevention research needs different strategies. As such, two types of family-focused modules need to be developed to supplement existing HIV prevention models. First, women who maintain contact with family members should be coached in ways that ensure that this experience adds value to the risk reduction process, rather than increasing risky behavior during times of stressful family interactions. Second, other women who no longer have contact with their family may need help processing feelings associated with being isolated from family members, as they may be participating in high risk behavior to numb the pain associated with family abandonment and isolation.

In addition, a special HIV prevention module needs to be developed for women who report having been sexually abused by a family member. Many women in this study lacked access to counseling, and have coped by suppressing their childhood sexual abuse. Moreover, many of these women are subjected to facing their abusers at family gatherings and are expected to "forgive and forget" to keep the family together. This ultimately results in them believing that they lack power to negotiate or communicate safer sex situations, as perceived powerlessness continues to haunt them from suppressed childhood sexual trauma.

Chapter 4

Intimate Relationships in the Rough

Me and him never used a condom 'cause I satisfied him and he satisfied me. And we didn't have no reason to go nowhere else and do nothing. So if it was just like in between us, we didn't have to wear no condom.

Karen, a 38-year-old crack cocaine and heroin user

HIV prevention research has effectively pinpointed women's HIV risk as tied to having one or more distinct types of sexual partners, including paying partners, casual partners, and intimate or steady partners (Amaro and Raj, 2000; DeCarlo and Quirk, 1998; Misovich, Fisher, and Fisher, 1997; Kane and Mason, 1992). Research has confirmed that in general, women are able to negotiate safer sex with paying and casual partners, albeit with varying degrees of success over time. However, research findings continue to report that high-risk women either do not want to use condoms with their intimate partners or their intimate partners will not use them (El-Bassel et al., 2001; Amaro and Raj, 2000).

In applying a black feminist perspective toward understanding unique experiences among black women at risk for HIV, this chapter examines five stages of intimate partner relationships identified by the women. A more in-depth analysis of women's intimate partner relationships is important in developing the next generation of HIV prevention interventions targeting high-risk heterosexual women that focus on helping women address their unique HIV needs at specific points along the life course of an intimate relationship (El-Bassel et al., 2001; Fullilove et al., 1990).

As heterosexual women's risk for HIV heightened, a dominant gender script emerged that instructs these women to avoid unprotected sex by insisting that every partner use a condom every time (Amaro and Raj, 2000; DeCarlo and Quirk, 1998; Misovich, Fisher, and Fisher, 1997; Kane and Mason, 1992). While this script has been relatively effective among women in negotiating condom use among their paying and casual partners, it has been less effective in intimate partner relationships. This chapter examines the meaning of intimate relationships in these women's lives, as well as the life course stages of women's relationships with intimate partners. Specifically, this study on women's intimate relationships focuses on the strategies women use across the life course of their intimate partner relationships to minimize their risk for HIV infection, while at the same time maximizing the emotional and financial benefits sought from their partners.

The inquiry into women's intimate relationships was perhaps the most complicated and complex part of this HIV prevention program. Unlike the other dilemmas these women faced, such as drug use, chronic unemployment, homelessness, motherhood, and lack of education, issues surrounding intimate relationships and one's risk for HIV are topics I have in common with the women. In fact, the conversations about intimate relationships with black men were similar to those I have with my own mainstream girlfriends as we struggle in trying to balance our needs for emotional and economic security with the need to be empowered and heard as strong black women capable of taking care of ourselves. Black women across class lines can relate to the perceived and real issues surrounding the pool of eligible black men (Wilson, 1996; Kline, Kline, and Oken, 1992). Clearly, instructing black women to insist that every partner use a condom every time further complicates relationships because black women want to trust their partners and condoms serve as a symbol of distrust (O'Leary and Wingood, 2000; Sherman, Gielen, and McDonnell, 2000; Moore, Harrison, and Doll, 1994). Moreover, many wish to procreate with intimate partners and a rigourous adherence to condom use with every partner every time will hinder procreation.

At first glance, the women in this study appeared to mirror my girlfriends, who typically display an outward level of high self-esteem relative to their choices in general, but are actually much more vulnerable in their intimate relationship choices. However, as I immersed myself in the narratives, I discovered that the structural context of poverty and social isolation makes a huge difference in the way in which I discuss intimate relationship issues with middle-class black women. While I was looking for perspectives we had in common, the structural constraints that high-risk women who are drug users, sex-workers, chronically unemployed, or caring for minor children grapple with as part of their everyday life makes it very difficult—but not impossible—to build a common solution for all black women at risk for HIV relative to our intimate partner relationships.

OVERVIEW OF THE FIVE STAGES OF INTIMATE PARTNER RELATIONSHIPS

The women in this study described their intimate partner relationships as being in one of five stages, consisting of the courtship, commitment, conflict, compromise, and conclusion stages. I refer to these stages collectively as the "life course of intimate relationships." Each stage is described in detail in the following sections of this chapter.

Figure 4.1, a conceptual framework of the five stages of intimate partner relationships, provides the conceptualization of the key stages of intimate partner relationships. Each stage is characterized by the extent of condom use and the level of trust women associate with each stage. The level of trust that women place in their intimate partners at key stages in a relationship is typically used as an explanation for why condoms are used and not used (Worth, 1989). The trust women have or do not have in their intimate partners may serve as a motivator or barrier in getting women to negotiate condom use with their

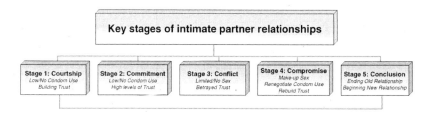

FIGURE 4.1. A conceptual framework of the five stages of intimate partner relationships.

intimate partners (Pulerwitz, Gortmaker, and DeJong, 2000). The stages associated with changes are further complicated by intimate partner violence and the threat of violence.

HIV prevention researchers must be open to a black feminist perspective that distinguishes between the "private" and "public" sex lives of high-risk women. Black women are more apt to discuss their public sex lives with paying and casual partners. However, when it comes to their emotional relationships, many black women learn to hide their self-defined standpoints from the dominant group. This is particularly the case as it relates to being in relationships with black men that the HIV prevention intervention community has labeled as the black woman's enemy within the context of HIV infection. At the same time, we must use culturally appropriate strategies for helping black women own the epidemiology data that state that black women are primarily infected by black men. I argue in this chapter that the key is to pinpoint risk within stages of a typical relationship and empower women to see how their risks change over the life course of an intimate relationship.

THE COURTSHIP STAGE

The courtship phase is characterized as the time to build trust, and because women perceive their partners to be "innocent until proven guilty," many do not ask their partners to use condoms while building trust and anticipating some level of economic stability. Although women in the Rough described having sexual intercourse with new intimate partners as early as the first night or within the first three weeks into the relationship, most women simply did not recall discussing condom use as part of the courtship stage. Instead, conversations during the courtship centered on intimate dating histories with others in the Rough, sources of income, and association with various drug-using networks. Some women said they use condoms only during the courtship phase if they know their partner is still dating other women. However, if a partner is able to convince a woman he is only intimate with her, then she will not insist on condom use. Karen highlights the complexities associated with trying to implement HIV prevention among women in the courtship stage with their intimate partners. She has been dating her current intimate partner for approximately seven years and provides a glimpse of the HIV-risk women encounter during the courtship stage.

> Me and my partner never use condoms. When I meet a guy, I'm a relationship lady. I ain't with that one night stand thang. I find out all about the person I mate with and we go on from there. But if it's something I don't like about you, then I'm just going to tell you I don't even think we should go any further. But the guy I'm with now, we been together seven years. But if I felt a need to or any other reason to wear [condoms], I would use them. But, we always have kept them in our bedroom and around. But, we never had used them for seven years we been together. So far, so good, no herpes or whatever. I ain't caught nothing, so I just never know what I would do without a li'l luck . . . The first time with him I think I should have. We had been talking 'bout two, three weeks, then that heated night came one night. In the heat of the night, boy, I tell you. I say, "damn I should have used a condom really. 'Cause hell, I don't know when he leave here what else he gone go out there and do, or what he been doing 'fore he got here."

As Karen explains, just as with others, high-risk women are seeking open and honest relationships in their choices for intimate partners. However, as with mainstream couples, individuals do not provide the details of their dating histories and risk factors during the courtship stage. So, even if the women had a list of all the right questions and subjects to bring up during the courtship stage as a way to address their HIV prevention needs, they would still be at the mercy of the male to respond truthfully. In this case, Karen uses the process of "reflecting back" on her lack of condom use with her partner from the beginning of the relationship. "Reflecting back" helped Karen to make sense of how her lack of knowledge about her intimate partner's sexual behavior prior to meeting her, as well as individuals he may have been having sex with during the same period they were having sex, left her vulnerable to the spread of HIV.

In examining women's narratives concerning the courtship stage, I discovered the issues and concerns women have as they enter new relationships. For the most part, women discussed how their choices of who to begin intimate partner courtships with centers on the potential male partner's ability to provide money or drugs from the outset of the relationship. Despite its effect on women's HIV prevention, what is less discussed or known is the man's expectations in return for the resources he brings to the relationship. Erica provided an example of how women may assert their needs to a potential intimate partner.

> I been knowed him from the neighborhood. He had kept on asking me, "Hey black girl, when you gone get with me?" I say, when your pocket get right. They call him Cadillac 'cause he got a Cadillac. So one evening it was about four o'clock. It was pouring down raining and I was making my way from down in the trap, and I was trying to walk fast up the hill. He turned at the corner, and he was like, you need a ride or something? I said, "no I'm almost home now." He talking about, who at your house; don't have me taking you home and no man shooting all out the door. I say, don't nobody live in my house but me and my mother and my sister. He like, damn so can I come to your house sometime? I say, I don't know about that. He dropped me off at the house. Well he was about to drop me off at the house, but he didn't want to drop me off. He didn't want to leave. He like, can we smoke in there? I say yeah, but I really don't like to 'cause I just don't feel comfortable smoking in our house 'cause it's my dead grandmama house. She died right in there . . . So I told him yeah. So we went and got some [dope] and we went in the house. He said, it's y'all in this big ole' house by yourself? I say, yeah just me and my sister, and my mother. I say, well my mother never here. He like, so what time she coming home? I say, she not coming here tonight she over to my aunt's house. [He asked] can I hang out over here for a li'l while? I'm like, buddy what you getting at? What you up too? Talking about, well I'm just trying to tell you li'l black girl I like you man. I told him I dig his big bens [money] in your pocket. He talking about, you ain't all that. I ain't got to be all that, I say, but all that I am, that's what I am. And that's what it's gone be. You can't just get me high. 'Cause I can get myself high. So I pulled out my own dope on him, and that tripped him out.

As Erica has articulated, while it is important for her to know she is in a relationship with a man who can provide money and access to drugs, she prides herself on being an independent woman. Erica and other women appeared to be less conscious of how men benefit from being in relationships with women who use crack cocaine. Cadillac has no house of his own; in return for the resources Erica needs from him in the relationship, he needs a safe place to smoke crack cocaine, engage in sexual intercourse, and sleep. He works as a valet parking attendant in the upscale area of Buckhead known for fine dining and upscale partying, and has a crack-related job of driving drug dealers around to run errands in and out of town. Men like Cadillac who are directly or indirectly linked to the crack economy as users and service providers, as well as having a full-time job with a constant cash flow via tips, are highly sought after as intimate partners in the Rough. Despite the flow of cash, Cadillac has not established himself as the head of household; instead, he moves constantly between the homes of family members and girlfriends. As Erica recalled, Cadillac seeks out women like her who can provide him a place to stay or a safe place to do drugs away from the crack house scene.

Women entering the courtship stages of intimate relationships do so within the context of gender role ideology that permeates our society. Historically, women have been pressured by key socializing institutions to be in committed relationships in ways that are different from how men are socialized to behave toward their intimate partners. Our religious, family, and economic institutions in particular reinforce the idea that women should commit and submit to intimate partners under even the toughest of circumstances and situations. In this way, the high-risk women in this study seek intimate partners as a way of having achieved mainstream relationship norms. Paradoxically, as women attempt to adhere to gender norms of intimate relationships during the courtship stage, they actually increase their risk for HIV (Sobo, 1995; Worth, 1989).

THE COMMITMENT STAGE

The commitment stage involves high levels of trust, as women believe they are in a monogamous relationship (Quina et al., 2000; Sobo, 1995). For most of these women, this can begin as early as a few days after meeting during the courtship stage or a few months into the courtship stage. The point is women tend to perceive themselves to be in committed relationships relatively early and may commit sooner than their male partners in hopes that the men will quickly follow their lead in being committed. Once relationships enter the commitment phase, some couples may move in together and attempt to set up household living and responsibility along traditional gender lines.

Carmen married her high school sweetheart and has two grown sons and four grandchildren. For the first eighteen years of the marriage, Carmen had a sense of stability through welfare, food stamps, public housing, and Medicaid. Once the boys were grown, she lost access to these government-sponsored programs, but was able to secure disability.

> We been together thirty-three years. Every time he hit he always get his own needle and use his own needle. But like if he was going to go do something with somebody, both the needles got to be new. But he gonna do his own stuff. They'll buy it up, but he's gonna pull his own up through his clean needle. I've been around and seen him do that. But I hope he don't be doing it behind my back; using nobody else needles. But I don't believe he would. Because he know what kind of chance he be taking with that AIDS. A lot of people got it from shooting dope too. A lot of heroin; a lot of them done died from it; shooting dope . . . We don't never have no sex . . . Well shit, it been so long honey I don't have no desire for it . . . To be truthful I really don't; so he don't neither. . . . No. Because I really wanted to know, you know, 'cause I hadn't messed around since he was in jail . . . he did about a year.

By all accounts, a thirty-three-year marriage is a long-term commitment, and to get this couple to practice safe sex seems next to impossible, despite their heightened risk for HIV due to both of them being heavy heroin users. Moreover, Carmen is convinced that they do not put each other at risk either by sharing dirty needles or having sex outside the relationship. She insists that she often observes Mark using his own clean needles. In addition, she rationalizes that because she doesn't desire to have sex, then neither does Mark.

Pamela's husband has helped her recover from a twenty-year crack cocaine and heroin habit. She provided a glimpse into everyday life of trying to maintain a committed intimate relationship with a non-using partner. His role in this case amounts to that of a committed codependent.

> Me and my husband went walking and stuff 'cause I told him that monkey on my back. And he know when I get fidgety, he say, come on let's go. He even took off work . . . I was married, but my husband didn't know I was turning dates then. He knows now . . . The little money my husband make, he don't make a whole lot either and he's putting back so that we can get us another place.

Frankie has been in a committed relationship with her intimate partner for over twenty years. Like many of the women who have intimate partners, Frankie is aware of her limitations in getting her partner to use condoms; therefore her safe sex strategy is to be sure she insists that all of her paying partners use condoms. In her mind, this way if she tests HIV positive she can trace her infection to unprotected sex with her intimate partner. She recalls her feelings and thoughts after taking an HIV test.

> I was positive that I didn't have AIDS because I hadn't put myself at risk to be able to get it. But if it would've came, it would have been through my husband. If he was out messing around in the streets. But I still say, I don't even put him at that risk. We been together twenty years and he all my children daddy. We was together when I didn't do [crack cocaine]. So he know me.

Frankie appears to be unsure as to whether her partner has unprotected sex with others in the street, but she remains confident that she doesn't put him at risk. She does turn tricks as a way to supply her drug habit without taking money from the family household. In addition, Frankie knows she could benefit from going into a residential drug treatment facility, but has refused to leave her husband. She describes her dilemma of trying to figure out how to benefit from a drug treatment program and maintain her twenty-year relationship, given the rules and regulations governing contact with intimate partners among typical drug treatment facilities. I asked her how long she would remain in the drug treatment center if she decided to go.

Six months. That's a long time. I'm sitting here and I'm telling you, but I'll be lying to myself and them to say that I can do it and I know I got other plans. Which might be wrong or might be right. But I ain't gonna be able to leave my children. Even though that's they daddy, he got to work. He can deal with my two boys 'cause they big boys. He can deal with them, if I was in prison he had to do it 'cause he have done it before. But I don't want to leave my girls. They need me. They need they mama for the motherly things that I have to do for them. That mean a lot and they need me. I don't know what I'm gonna do. I really don't. But I know I gotta find me a job. And I'm gone find something to do. And I'm just thankful for my husband that do provide for us . . . I was thinking like, well they say you get to come out, go to work. And I can be coming by my house, checking on my house. Which I wanna do it 'cause I really do [attend drug treatment].

Frankie is faced with going to a drug treatment facility where she is not guaranteed financial or emotional support versus remaining in a relationship where she has a twenty-year track record with an intimate partner who has proven himself as a stable and consistent provider for her and the children. Thus, Frankie is trying to find a way to maintain the relationship while meeting the requirements of the drug treatment program. However, Frankie sees drug treatment as a barrier to her economic and emotional stability. To be clear, intimate partners are viewed as enablers or hindrances in recovery, and many drug treatment programs strongly recommend that participants adhere to rules of not contacting partners in the early stages of recovery. In this way, women like Frankie conclude that drug treatment will actually decrease her level of stability and support as opposed to serve as a resource for lowering her risk for HIV.

Several women maintain committed relationships during their own as well as their partner's jail time. Ka-Ka, for example, who served three years for drug dealing, maintained a ten-year relationship with her intimate partner. After he completed his sentence he joined Ka-Ka in Atlanta a few months after she left the Rough for drug rehabilitation. Ka-Ka describes how she immediately began having unprotected sex with her intimate partner after he moved to Atlanta.

I want to terminate this pregnancy . . . He just came down here. We was distant. We've always been together though. I got him a job at the pie factory. I used to work there. We used to sell drugs, too. He was locked up. Both of us was locked up . . . I had done three years. I got busted back home . . . Everybody get their chance to shine. We was rolling. I wanted to try to keep him home because he was messing around on me. And I was using. I wasn't looking like nothing. But I messed up, because they was watching my house . . . I had to go to prison, and he took good care of me.

Over the course of my fieldwork, Erica and Cadillac's relationship moved from the courtship to the commitment stage. Erica, who knows from past relationships that these types of arrangements are tenuous, maintains her permanent residency with her family. When I met up with Erica after her intervention, during the conversation she mentioned that she thought she was pregnant by Cadillac. Erica describes a typical day in the commitment stage of her relationship with Cadillac in the Rough.

Basically when I get up, I feed my baby. I go back to sleep. Might sex a li'l while, and go back to sleep until he get ready to go to work. When he get up and go to work, that's when I get up and go home. But we don't get high everyday, and I'm glad about that. I feel better about that, 'cause I was burned out. I didn't have no strength. But now I take me a vitamin everyday. I love him. I mean me and him get along great. He be like two hundred dollars strong when he come home. That's after he pay the club. He have like one hundred and seventy dollars when he come home. He automatically fixing to give me twenty dollars that's going in my pocket. That's for whatever. That ain't for the cigarettes. That is my little allowance I guess. Then he gone go around the corner, he gone pay his little tab off. He might owe the dope man around the corner. We got one man around the corner that work the graveyard shift. Mr. Q-Stick sell beer, liquor, dope, everything. You get one rock, a pack of cigarettes, a beer maybe, that's twenty dollars. So by the time he get home and give me twenty dollars that leave him at one hundred and fifty dollars. Then he go around to the dope dealer and give him twenty dollars. That leave him like one hundred and thirty dollars. I say he'll spend that thirty dollars buying us something to smoke. Then he'll spend five dollars and buy him a half-pint or a cocktail for the night. I don't drink. So, when he get back to the house it depends on what day it is 'cause if he pay his uncle for living there something like ten dollars a day.

As Erica describes their daily lives, even though they don't have a place of their own, it is very clear that during the commitment stage, relationships take on the norms and role expectations typically associated with married couples in our society. Cohabitation has proven to be a difficult task for most women in the Rough, as they tend to couple with men, who like themselves, lack personal stability and access to the basic resources needed to maintain a household over longer periods of time. Nevertheless, there are some couples that, despite drug use and lack of stable housing and employment, remain committed to the relationship. To be sure, not all of these women are in relationships with men who use drugs. However, what became clear as I inquired about the types of drugs used is that women did not classify drinking beer and liquor or smoking marijuana as drug use. I learned that when women stated their intimate partners didn't use drugs, I needed to ask specifically about alcohol and marijuana use. The clarity was not needed because women were trying to hide their partner's usage patterns, but because within the Rough, those who drink alcohol or smoke marijuana, but do not use crack, cocaine, or heroin, are not considered drug users.

Allison articulates the complexity of condom use during the commitment stage of intimate partner relationships. In exchange for taking care of women financially, men expect to have sexual intercourse without a condom. To be sure, women also see condom use as a barrier in intimate relationships. I asked Allison what would happen in her relationship if she asked her intimate partner of four years to use a condom.

Well, I think I may have to find somewhere else to go . . . I want to keep Leroy. Leroy gone take care of me. Sometimes if I wanna smoke one hundred, two hundred, three hundred dollars worth of dope a day he can't give me that much money. I don't take no bill money. I might get about five to ten dollars from him in two or three days. I might say, Baby, give me some money. I don't get his hard-working money for me to go out to smoke dope. Now, I'd go out and turn tricks to pay bills sometimes instead going out and smoking it up. I just go to the rent man and hand him the money or go to the grocery store and buy up all the groceries I can buy. A junkie can't have money in their hand.

Allison prides herself on supplying her drug habit through protected sex work without taking money from the household. However, most women are unable to effectively keep their household expenses separate from their drug money. It is not uncommon for women and their partners in the Rough to be evicted from fragile attachments to housing and sometimes find themselves homeless as they seek alternative living arrangements. Martha's narrative provides a glimpse of what ultimately happens to women in intimate relationships who are unable to maintain their living arrangements. Martha's partner of six years smokes crack with her, and unable to maintain, they smoked up their rent money. Martha discussed how she and her boyfriend of five years have remained committed as a homeless couple.

I lost my room . . . that was making me smoke more and more and I had started getting kind of depressed. People say something to me, I use to just want to go off on them. I thought everybody was picking on me at that time. But, I think I was getting depressed by not having nowhere to stay . . . I had me a Jeep and I had cover and stuff back there. I'll sleep out there. Some nights some friends would say, hey you ain't going to sleep out there in that cold, come on in. They'll let me come in and sleep. But I just got tired of that. . . . He was outside too. See, he get disability too, and we both be messing up. 'Cause it's hard for two drug addicts to try and keep the other one strong. That's just like the blind leading the blind. So, I couldn't hardly help him and he couldn't help me. 'Cause I was constantly smoking and he was constantly smoking . . . He's forty-five. But he don't need to use and I don't either; but he got Parkinson disease. The Parkinson already make you shake. He smoke that stuff and try to stand up and sometimes he fall slam down. And that scares me to death. By being around him and see how he act when he smoking. I'm going to quick smoking. 'Cause I tell him all the time, I'm fixing to quit smoking this stuff 'cause it's making me scared.

Women described experiences during their commitment phase that I term "coming and going." The process of coming and going is characterized by time spent apart during a committed relationship. This time apart can be self-initiated or systemically imposed. Self-initiated "coming and going" can be either the man or woman leaving the relationship for some period of time, and can be with or without warning. Coming and going during the commitment stage can be as short as a few hours to cool off after a heated argument—something that is common, even encouraged, in mainstream relationships as a conflict resolution tactic. However, because of the influence of chronic drug use that characterizes these women's relationships in the Rough, drug binges can result in women being away from an intimate partner for days or even weeks at a time. Still other women take to the streets to escape more severe domestic violence situations that escalate well past arguing to pushing and shoving.

Systemically imposed coming and going generally results when one or both individuals go to jail, or are court ordered to drug treatment, or it can be job related. However, most coming and going among women and men involved in drug using and dealing is a result of serving jail time (Comfort et al., 2000). For example, Johnsie and her partner go to jail periodically and at different times for petty theft and breaking public ordinance rules. Because they are both homeless, they must reconnect on the streets after one or both of them are released from jail sentences ranging on average from two to ninety days; although it is not uncommon for repeat offenders of misdemeanors to serve twelve to eighteen months for violating probation. In fact, when I was hanging out with Johnsie, she mentioned she had just been released from jail and that she was waiting on her partner who had also recently been released.

Anthony just got out of jail Monday. He went to jail the day before I did for a can of beer. I'm like, I'm getting out and you going in. I still haven't seen him and don't want to. I just want to know if he going to take the time from whatever he doing to stop and look for me like I'm looking for him. And when we do see each other it's going be like hey, what's up, how much you got?

Johnsie tries to play tough, as if she only wants money from Anthony. However, she equates his action of not looking for her after being released from jail with not caring about her and disrespecting their relationship. Women in the Rough also see maintaining relationships while men are in jail for longer periods of time as a normal part of intimate relationships with men in the Rough, and they may not fully understand the ways in which reuniting with men after they have spent time in jail ranks as a high-risk sexual encounter.

What may be even harder to address is the fact that women believe their men are faithful when they are incarcerated, and they have countless letters and phone calls confirming their beliefs. Janice explains how high-risk women take on the caregiving role to men coming out of jail, helping them reestablish themselves after serving jail sentences.

> I been with Buster since 1996. But Lord knows I want to end me and Buster. We cool and all but I want to end it. I know one time he had did sixteen months. But it was seventeen [months] since we had been apart 'cause I was locked up for a month. Then when I got out that month, he got out Christmas Eve. He came from Gwinnett County and had on his getting high stuff. He got broke and can't talk. He be like a lost cause, just like a new baby on the street. He always come to me when he get to that point. He wait 'til everything gone and helpless then come find me and put the burden on my shoulder. I'm in the street too.

While some women are at risk with partners who come and go as part of serving jail sentences, others have partners who are away as part of their job. Truck drivers and construction workers who find work in nearby states or rural counties in Georgia are typically characterized as men with good jobs among women in the Rough. Mattie's partner is one such man who comes and goes as part of his job as a truck driver. Mattie explains that she likes the monetary benefits of having a gainfully employed man; however, she claims she doesn't have sex with him because she doesn't know who he has sex with while out on the road.

> Don't come think you fixing to play in here naked. You can't play house here. You might better squeeze it to death with five of them over there. I say, I don't know nothing about you when you go up and down that road.

Ingrid described herself as the one that comes and goes. Her partner is the stable one. She comes to the Rough to do drugs and prostitute. She gets stuck some nights and can't get home. She goes to jail and he gets her out.

> I been with him twelve years. He's retired from the Army and stuff. He ain't that old, I'm forty. I just had some sleep last night. I really don't sleep when I done been over here. I slept all day and all night yesterday . . . he think something, but he just won't say nothing.

Perhaps the couples in the commitment stage have the most promise for couple-centered HIV prevention albeit if both individuals acknowledge their commitment to the other person. Typically, HIV prevention programs targeting heterosexual couples primarily do so by targeting women; however, it is clear from these women's accounts of their committed partnerships that couples need to share in the responsibility of HIV prevention, much in the same way they share other responsibilities in the relationship (El-Bassel et al., 2001). To date, very few HIV-risk reduction interventions address intimate heterosexual partners as couples committed to the long-term stability and health of their relationship with each other (El-Bassel et al., 2001). Not only is the dominant safe sex script overly narrow in general for women, it is shortsighted in terms of a women's desire to be in committed, loving relationships where they share uninhibited sexual intimacy (Bowleg, Belgrave, and Reisen, 2000; Grinstead, Zack, and Faigeles, 1999; Gomez and Marin, 1996). For this reason, the commitment stage is generally a time when couples are highly likely to engage in unprotected sex no matter the initial rules for condom use. Even more complicated is the idea that some women are in committed relationships with men they know to be in "concurrent commitments," in which they are intimately tied to several women. To be fair, some women in the Rough were in concurrent commitments as well. This concept is discussed more in depth as a part of the compromise stage.

THE CONFLICT STAGE

As with any intimate partner relationship, women in the Rough who remain committed over a period of time will face conflict at various points. The conflict stage is marked by some event or series of events that generally manifest as a betrayal of trust. Also, during this time sexual intercourse between committed individuals may decrease or cease altogether. Moreover, "heightened conflict" in which individuals may get to a boiling point—but still not a breaking point—could also mark a time when individuals try to justify sex outside the intimate relationships. However, conflict in intimate partner relationships between drug-using couples is very complex in general, as conflict often occurs with overlapping dynamics and processes. For drug using and codependent couples, conflict in relationships is described on one level as involving arguing about drugs and money as well as ongoing accusations of cheating and lying. Intimate partner conflict is further complicated by unresolved past issues that resurface during a current conflict. As the women described it, for the most part, at the base of most of their conflicts with intimate partners are underlying factors such as not trusting men, not feeling respected by them, and not believing the men are honest or are listening to their concerns. Erica describes how conflict over drugs causes relationship problems.

> And I hate when he drink that liquor. I don't like people when they drink. He just turn into a drunk hell. I don't drink and I don't like drunk character. He be like, baby you'll do this, just like he's just helpless or something. He want me to do everything. I be like, when am I gonna be able to sit down and take a hit of my shit. You don't want me to be out in the daytime or at night while you at work. You want me to stay at home 'til you get home from work 'cause you can take care of your woman. I come home. I got to sit there and wait on him then. I'm just like this. I serve my man. I don't care. Now I hook it up. The only thing I don't be with that liquor part. You gone fix your own drink, pour your own trouble. I cut the crack for him. I sat our pipes out for him. He spoiled. He just forget all about me. When it's my turn he be done found something else to ask me to do. I say, you are so selfish and so greedy. I'm not gone accept anymore from you than I'm willing to offer you. I ain't gone ask you for no more than you can ask me for. And if you can't live by that, partner you got to find you somebody else to live with. 'Cause you don't want me to go home.

Janice's example of intimate relationship conflict centers on her trying to get money for the couple's drugs and living expenses, but because her boyfriend is jealous, they often have disagreements that escalate into unhealthy conflict.

> It's like I'll catch some guys got some money. I'll tell them where I live if they worth coming there then I tell Buster. He'll get smart. What you want Janice for? I'll tell him if a guy knock on the door it's worth letting them in. We might be hungry or want some dope. And somebody knock on the door it be blessing. I'm doing all the work. I'm going to get the dope. I'm doing everything 'cause he helpless. Then the guy may want to stay there with him and give him the money and I say put your hustle down. He go and he say that ain't my style. Then he'll say well if you knock on the door or come home and a woman here don't get upset. I say cool you know I be serious.

During the conflict stage, domestic violence in intimate relationships continues to serve as a barrier in high-risk women's HIV prevention. Literature regarding HIV infection shows that there is a strong connection between HIV and domestic violence (Molina and Basinait-Smith, 1998; Kalichman et al., 1998). Further complicating the issues surrounding how to effectively address HIV prevention needs in the lives of women experiencing domestic violence is the fact that most of the women did not characterize themselves as victims of domestic violence, primarily because they fight back. In their mind, a victim of domestic violence is one who does not fight back. They describe themselves as fighting back and see some level of physical fighting as a normal part of the relationship. In fact, many women described themselves as the initiator or aggressor when it comes to domestic violence. Because they do not perceive themselves to be victims of domestic violence, they are less likely to call the police or to seek refuge in a domestic violence shelter. Allison describes how domestic violence is a daily part of these Rough relationships.

> Me and him got the fighting the other night. Me and him was fighting it out. He was trying to hold me down. I told him I was going to put him in jail. I ain't do it. He jumped on top. Nothing was sitting up there in my mouth but a set of balls. I bit his balls

and blood just running all out of him. Then I jumped up and I say, you won't come back.

When I first met Shanese, she described her intimate partner relationship as chaotic and filled with daily conflict. I began to think to myself, *How do you ask a woman who already is battling verbally and physically with her partner to raise the notion of condom negotiation?*

> What I go through in a day now, arguing . . . My baby-daddy. I'm tired . . . Taking me through a lot of changes [fist fighting] and drugs, but we'll smoke, and then I can't handle no more . . . He'll be thirty-two Sunday. And I cannot handle no more pressure. But it had got to the violent part, real, real violent . . . Him throwing, tearing up stuff and he don't know how to communicate. You can communicate about drugs, but you cannot communicate about our relationship. I have been with different mens, true enough, but in the relationship part I keep getting the same result. The up and down relationship. He said, Can I stop? But then, if you give me a chance, and I see that I got a man willing to stand by me all through thick and thin, I might change.

THE COMPROMISE STAGE

Some women compromise as a way to protect themselves from the escalation of verbal and physical conflict. The compromise stage is highly likely to include episodes of make-up sex with no condom use as a gesture toward recommitment and rebuilding trust that may have been lost or damaged during the conflict stage. During the compromise stage, however, women often sacrifice their own self-interests and concerns toward their protection against HIV infection. Women compromise because they believe that placing demands on their partners will in some way alter or damage the relationship. In essence, women who compromise in their relationship are following the dominant gender script that women should be submissive and silent in response to their intimate partner's needs.

The compromise stage is conceptualized as a time in a relationship when women abandon what they really want and value in a relation-

ship in order to keep an intimate partner. The things that they want
and value evolve around trust, respect, financial security, and monogamy. During the compromise stage women use various strategies and
tactics to minimize conflict and maximize the benefits of being in an
intimate relationship. Women discussed the aspects of their relationship that they compromise on, which impacts their risk for HIV infection. Women make sense of their decisions to compromise by stating
that the physical fights are not as violent as they once were. Other
women discussed how their partners provide the best way they can, in
a way that justifies why they resort to compromises rather than leave
the relationship. Even if some women gained a sense of empowerment to protect themselves—particularly if prior conflicts centered
on cheating—they may become emotionally vulnerable as it relates
to protecting themselves during the compromise stage. It is here they
develop a sense of complacency about HIV risk as they accept that
men cheat and lower their expectations to that of "he can cheat as long
as he doesn't give me a disease." Frankie provides her perspective on
how women make sense of why they compromise in long-term intimate relationships.

> I don't even worry about if he cheat. Just don't get no disease.
> 'Cause we done been together for so long, to that part don't even
> matter. We been together so long, he probably want something
> different. You know how mens is. So I don't even worry about
> that part. Who knows what this man might be doing when he
> ain't with me. 'Cause he ain't no perfect angel.

Women in the compromise stage provide accounts of their intimate
partner relationships that appear to fluctuate along a continuum of
pain and pleasure. For example, on the one hand, Sharon's partner had
inflicted so much emotional and physical pain on her that she was
actually contemplating suicide.

> I had wrote a letter about hurting myself. I can't remember from
> word to word. But I didn't let that guy just push me so much and
> I try to believe in him and he always let me down with my kids.
> He promised me he wasn't gonna put his hands on me and he
> broke that. I started breaking away from him.

Later, however, Sharon discussed the pleasure she derives from having make-up sex with her partner. According to Sharon, "He said that I wasn't never gonna leave that bed not satisfied . . . I had two kids before I had my first climax and when I did I thought I was having a heart attack . . . I thought sex was boring . . . But when I felt satisfied." It is clear from these two contrasting statements from Sharon on how easy it is to compromise in a relationship that can be very painful in one extreme and yet pleasurable at the other extreme.

It is not uncommon for women to strategize in terms of how to manage their needs during the compromise stage. For example, women learn to find other places to smoke their crack cocaine to avoid sharing with men they describe as "greedy" when it comes to drugs. Many women seek other places to avoid being sent out into the streets to turn tricks for more drugs. Martha explains how she manages to avoid her drug-using partner.

> Since I been on drugs, I don't have a sexual drive anymore. I don't even want sex that much. A lot of times for instance I have money and I go buy some dope. I leave my own place and go smoke by myself.

High-risk women enter and exit intimate partnerships more frequently, primarily due to a lack of adequate resources needed for long-term stability. Such inability of women's primary partners to provide financially has resulted in some women hedging their bets with "concurrent intimate partners," having one or more intimate partners at the same time. Women may decide to have more than one intimate partner, hence the phrase "concurrent partners," as opposed to "multiple partners," which has been used to signify multiple levels of partners. Multiple partnerships may exist on three levels, including paying, casual, and intimate/steady partners. Janice provides a definition of concurrent partners that may start out as categorized as a multiple partner.

> Mens that I know that really care about me and it's like four. I ain't really trying to be serious 'cause some of them smoke; half of them smoke. They care for me, deal with me. Imagine four men really care about you and they know what you going through, try to deal with you. You go to them, but it's some, they

try to get you to make a choice. But you lie about the rest of
them, saying, ain't nobody but you. But then the list adding on.
They want you to make a choice.

The primary distinction is that multiple partners are additive or lay-
ered, whereas concurrent partners are all considered intimate partners.
Concurrent partners may all believe they are the only one, whereas
multiple partners tend to know that there are other partners. For example, in traditional risk reduction programs women are asked about
their intimate partners, casual partners, and paying partners. However, there is no line of questioning that asks them to explain their risk
factors among several partners who may all be intimate partners.

Tosha provides a perspective on multiple-partners and the impact
they have on the spread of HIV. She continues to do sex work but she
will not carry condoms. She hides her sex work activities from her intimate partners as best she can, and thus relies on her paying partners
to have condoms. In Tosha's case her compromise tactic actually increases her risk for unprotected sex because she is now relying solely
on her paying sexual partners to (1) agree to use a condom and
(2) have a condom on them.

> I got an old man. I can't walk around with condoms. He will not
> hear that. We been together for four years now. You know him.
> I done got caught last night if you wanna know the truth. His ex-
> boss man called and he was like, what is he doing calling up here.
> I say, I guess he just call to see what you wanted. I say, I didn't
> call him.

Being in a relationship with married men is part of the compromise
stage as well. For example, Peaches admits she prefers older married
men who are looking for companionship outside of their marriage.
She describes the relationship.

> My friend I'm with now, I've been knowing him for twenty-
> seven years. But we been together since 1993. He brought me a
> long way. He picked me up knowing about my drug habits and
> everything. He just accepted me for who I was. Because he was
> a retired schoolteacher. And I always admired him for the way
> he carried himself. And he's eighteen years my senior. He got a

wife. That's the only person I deal with, because God gave me
the sense to realize that's the only person who gone stand by me.
He had stayed down to [the Hospital] with me for two days
'cause I fell in the bathtub . . . And he's so good that I don't want
to turn him loose. And he's not fixing to turn me loose . . . He
does everythang for me. He washed my clothes. He dried them.
He unpacked all one hundred and eleven of the boxes that we
took over there. He hung the drapes, the Venetian blinds. He
shampooed the carpet. He's out there now doing the lawn. He
buy the douche. He buy the soap. He buy the washing powder,
the bleach. I got TV in the bathroom, TV in kitchen. I say he is
too good to be true.

Shanté describes how she learned to cope with a cheating and a
violent partner as part of the compromise stage.

He used to be worser then, but it done calm down some. 'Cause
we used to fight a lot. We don't fight that much now 'cause I don't
argue back with him . . . But then we don't even be intimate no
more like we used too 'cause I don't know what he be doing out
there. 'Cause sometime he'll stay gone, so I don't even hardly
just trust being intimate with him. He work every day. Just be
out there and I don't know them women, he be riding in the car
and I just don't say nothing. 'Cause I know that's how a man
gone be. I say, well I sho' ain't fixing to be worried about him.

One of the reasons why women like Shanté describe their relationships with their intimate partners as relatively calm or not as bad as it
once was is because they are constantly comparing themselves to the
poor state of intimate partner relationships among other women in
the Rough. For example, Shanté knows her physical altercations are
not as severe as what Punkin experiences. Because Punkin's partner
is so publically violent and is often observed hitting, cursing, and
"snapping" on Punkin in full view of others in the Rough, many
women measure their violent encounters against Punkin's experiences. In my own observations, I too concluded that Punkin faces the
worse type of interaction with her intimate partner. She describes
how violence is very much a part of her everyday intimate partnership.

He like to fight. We don't fight like we used to . . . Last I seen y'all I had two pins in my jaw from fighting. The last time my jaw was broke . . . It's because of him that I'm out there . . . He don't send me out there just to turn tricks. We just get into a fight or something or he be like he don't want me to pack my bags and shit. He know what that consists of anyway . . . In a week, fights? Well physically we haven't got to any fights like that lately . . . Yeah. We got into an argument today.

THE CONCLUSION STAGE

There were ten women who left abusive or drug-using partners over the course of this ethnographic study. Jennifer was one such woman, and she describes how the relationship went through all the stages in the life course from courtship to conclusion.

He met me when we was dating and stuff. [Stage 1: Courtship]

I had really fell in love with that man. He had stop smoking dope and everything. I'm a good girl that need a good man. [Stage 2: Commitment]

But come to find, hey you doing the dirt. [Stage 3: Conflict]

When I started looking good and pretty, I was staying in the house. The lady downstairs say, she don't never come out the house. When he lay down and go to sleep, I had to lay beside him. He really didn't have too much trust in me. He always got to come and apologize about this and that; tell me 'bout his problem with other women. Call hisself trying to play with my mind and emotions. He was hitting me, beating me. He couldn't understand that's why I was out there on the street. I was walking up and down the street and stuff. [Stages 3 and 4: Conflict and Compromise]

I told him it's about me loving me and also me loving you too. . . , I told him, we gone be safe whether you like it or you don't. [Stage 3: Conflict]

He started going along [Stage 4: Compromise]

but then we broke up. [Stage 5: Conclusion]

As Jennifer's account of a recent intimate relationship confirms, HIV prevention messages must be appropriate for the stage the relationship is in. It is important to note that when Jennifer attempted to communicate with her partner about condom use after getting HIV counseling, her partner eventually broke off the relationship.

Jennifer went on to describe how he began hitting her and beating her because he couldn't understand why she was on the street, given that she lived with family. She described him as a man she met while on the street who smoked crack but has a good job mixing chemicals. His reactions to Jennifer's condom-use request confirms my earlier contention that men with jobs in an urban poor setting are less likely to adhere to any requests from women against their wishes. These men know that others perceive them to be good providers, and they tend to change partners rather than meet the demands of one woman. However, because Jennifer is family housed she could make the choice to break up with him. Women who depend on their steady partners for their livelihood are less likely to raise the issue in the first place.

I remember vividly the day one of the outreach workers brought Cynthia to the HIP House. By this time I had become an interventionist and Cynthia was assigned to me at random during her first visit. She was bleeding and had bruises in her face and chest area. She was crying in a whimpered tone. I was impressed that the outreach worker had convinced her to come to the HIP House in such a state because most women don't want to be seen in such pain. Cynthia described at length how she and her steady partner had fought for a year. She expressed wanting a way out, but had no place to go. While Cynthia returned home that day, we agreed that she would plan and execute an escape from this relationship. She returned for two more sessions at the HIP House and each time appeared stronger and more determined than the previous time. As I documented in her file, I observed an increased self-esteem during her intervention; I was not surprised when some eight months later during her qualitative interview she announced that she had left him four months earlier.

> I don't stay with him no more. I stay with my girlfriend. This was last year at the end of the year. He had got put out. When he got put out I left him. I quit running around and all I need is to just get me a job and I'll be alright.

Cynthia took advantage of his loss of stable housing as a time to escape. Even without a job or prospect for new living arrangements, Cynthia left her steady partner. She went on to say that she earns money by babysitting for some of the women in the community who have gone to work under the welfare reform mandate. She has no children of her own and expressed that child care would be temporary for her as she has no desire to mother other people's children.

While Cynthia was able to escape without further violence, Michelle's story provides a glimpse into the idea that some intimate partners turn violent when the women try to get out of the relationship.

> When I first met him it was on the trick style. And then his emotions and shit. He wanted to be my man, and he couldn't accept no. So for a year and a half I went through total hell. I mean he stalking. Where I stay at now in the rooming house, all my windows busted out. But see he locked up now for breaking and entering, terrorist threats, two counts of stalking . . . Because see he came through my bedroom window. And see I'm on top of the store. He got bound over with no bond. So it'll be some months before we even go back to court. I put on when I was in the courtroom. When the judge said bound over and bond remain the same. He was like, Yeah bitch I'm gone get out and I'm gone do this. Man I stood right there in front of that judge and cried. I say, You heard what he said? He gone get me, he gone get me. So I got a restraining order with two hundred feet. If he way up the street and I even recognize him he too close to me.

Women in the Rough expressed growing sick and tired of the negative consequences of their intimate relationships as the primary reason for exiting. Prior to actually ending the relationship, however, women undergo a process of "contemplating the conclusion" of the relationship. When I spoke with Martha, she described herself as being tired of drugs and was beginning to understand that if she really wanted to be drug free, she may have to end her six-year relationship with her current partner.

> Right now I'm tired. I'm tired of smoking. But sometimes I think about just telling him I got to go my own way. 'Cause I need to

get up off of dope and I don't think he going to stop smoking. Because when I say I don't want no dope today, he'll wanna send me out to get it and after I go out to get it, when I come back my mind done changed. I'm ready to smoke. Sometimes you got to separate from your, partner, your boyfriend, sometimes you got to separate to do what's best for you. And I kind of feel that I'm going to have to do that and I've been with him six years.

Clearly, abusive and controlling relationships take their toll on women's mental health. Near the conclusion of some relationships in which women have been severely abused, they may have thoughts of harming their intimate partners or themselves. Mona describes how easy it is to go from a domestic violence victim to fighting back.

He just keep pushing me. What do I care about setting your ass on fire? I'm serious. I love the smell of gasoline.

While most women described themselves as making the decisions to leave, Lisa painted a picture of how some men initiate the close of a relationship. Within the context of a high-risk environment, Lisa's boyfriend would be characterized as a good man. She has known him since high school, he has a good job and provided for her and her family before he fathered her third child. Lisa admitted to being stressed out due to a number of issues including intimate partner abandonment.

I done kicked him to the curb. I ain't going tell no lie. I didn't kick him to the curve. It just one day he up and left and said I'll be back and I ain't seen him since a couple of months. Matter of fact almost a year. But we knew each other when we was teenagers. When we was young we used to go together. And so we call ourself reuniting back together. He was saying, I'll be back. He was working. He does air conditionings and heatings and stuff like that.

Sabrina ended a violent relationship as part of her HIV prevention goals. She describes how her risk reduction counselor helped her understand how the relationship was not beneficial.

The dude I used to go with used to jump on me, beat on me. I don't go with him no more. I had him locked up. And he did the time. I seen him about two to three days ago, but I don't speak to him. He was trying to bring me down. He was smoking. He was doing the snort, whatever they call it. So [my HIV prevention counselor] was saying get away from him. He trying to bring you down. And I listen to her and I talk to her. As I talked to her about the problem, she told me I could be somebody once I get rid of him. I'm like, she's telling me the truth. I need to be somebody. I need to dress. I'm not no bad-looking person. And I started listening to her and it happened. I got rid of him and it was like a relief. It feel good and then I was like, now I won't really worry about no dope. I got me a good job. I can come home. I can buy me clothes. I can get my hair fixed. I can do lots of things. And I started going to the club and taking me pictures, having my hair braided up, dressing up.

In classic co-dependency theory, Sabrina implies that she only continued using drugs because she had a steady partner who used them. Many drug-using women often give their drugs and/or money to drug-using male partners. As Sabrina expressed, many of the interventionists, including myself, took every opportunity to let the women know they were worthy of decent relationships. All of us were careful, however, not to provoke the men in these women's lives, some of whom would be waiting right on the front porch of the HIP House during the intervention. While I never condoned the violence, I always wondered, given these men's own bouts with structured oppression and personal depression, would a steady partner session have helped these couples? Such an approach to intervention would be an application of what some black feminists call womanism, which is a form of feminism espoused by black women to acknowledge the inequality that black men suffer along with black women at the hands of structural domains of power. Although Sabrina was able to conclude a violent intimate relationship, in less than six months she was in a relationship with another drug-using unemployed man in the Rough. As a risk reduction strategy, however, she did not allow this new man to move in.

He don't work. He's scared child support gonna find out he working and took all his money. I told him it's best for him to get another job. He gone try to do construction work. We been to-gether since last year November. I ain't gone let him move in with me. I can't support them. I doing better to support myself.

Lisa has taken on a harder attitude toward new relationships than did Sabrina. Lisa was hurt and now vows not to be in another intimate relationship. She believes this stance will protect her emotionally.

> I'm scared . . . Because I don't want another him. The little one. I don't want no 'nother him. So, I just rather just take it as I go. If I meet somebody, I'll like you and all that. I'll do like the men do. I like you and all that, get me a rubber and do it and bye bye. 'Cause women have their needs too. But I'm not with that. This not going there no more. I don't want another him.

The findings from this chapter reject several bodies of existing knowledge concerning high-risk women's risk for HIV. First, research-ers grounded in social psychology theoretical frameworks suggest that women suffer from a lack of perceived power stemming directly from low self-esteem (Bowleg, Belgrave, and Reisen, 2000). Still, other researchers have argued that inner-city women have low expecta-tions for the men in their lives (Sharpe, 2001). My research suggests that the women actually have very high expectations of their intimate partners, but are unable to hold the men accountable for their actions. What I did unravel is that women's perspectives of their relationships are marked often by inconsistencies between what they believe and how they behave, primarily due to their limited prospects for men who value what they value—and not the fact that the women don't have values.

The dominant HIV prevention script of condom use with every part-ner narrows high-risk women's choices of safe sex options because they don't actually use condoms, but rather must convince someone else to use them. As revealed among the women, condom use with inti-mate partners across the life course of the relationship can be problem-atic on several dimensions. First of all, condom use in heterosexual relationships continues to manifest as a strategy that women must con-vince men to adhere to in much the same way birth control has been so-cially constructed as the woman's responsibility. Second, asking men to use condoms can lead to increased rates and severity of domestic violence. Finally, women see condom use as associated with short-term sexual encounters that lack emotional intimacy. HIV prevention programs must consider how condom use with intimate partners is rejected, and seek longer term safer sex solutions that view the couple as having a real chance at balancing gender power, making collaborative safer sex choices, and having commitment to the relationship over a longer period of time. Specifically, couples could benefit from conflict resolution and more effective communication techniques.

HIV prevention research indicates that risks associated with intimate relationships places women at higher risk for HIV in comparison to casual and paying partners. These women's accounts of the dynamics associated with intimate partner relationships suggest that condom use is not highly desirable among the women themselves. Instead, these high-risk women want what mainstream women want in their intimate relationships—trust, financial security, honesty, communication, respect, and appreciation for their caregiving and/or homemaking, as well as monogamy. As such, it is clear from these women's accounts that basic HIV/AIDS strategies centered on condom use do not translate easily into intimate couple relationships. In these women's estimation, they want both parties to be fully committed to a monogamous relationship so that condom use will not be necessary.

HIV prevention strategies and tactics for women who are at different stages and phases in their intimate partner relationships are limited. Simply telling women to tell their intimate partners to use a condom everytime may be unrealistic if it is in conflict with other competing goals. Depending on a woman's own perception of the stage of her intimate partner relationship, she may need different HIV prevention messages.

PRINCIPLES TO GUIDE A COUPLES-CENTERED HIV PREVENTION INITIATIVE

A partner centered HIV prevention program addressing the dilemmas of black women and their intimate partners will need to be grounded in a womanist theoretical perspective because it takes into account how both genders within the African-American community experience racism and poverty in ways that increase their chances for

HIV infection (Nyamathi and Stein, 1997). As this chapter examined five stages of high-risk women's intimate partner relationships, it is clear that HIV prevention researchers must develop more relevant modules to address women and their intimate partners' risks for HIV infection. HIV prevention programs can enhance their inquiry into intimate relationships as a first step toward more effective HIV prevention messages. A more thorough assessment of one's intimate relationship should include strategies to determine the number of intimate partners women have at any given point. Second, determine which stage women perceive themselves to be in with their intimate partners. Once women pinpoint what stage they are in, then the HIV prevention counselor can focus on specific HIV risks and protection issues.

Women talked tough about their intimate partner relationships, and without digging deeper, prevention counselors might conclude that the women have more personal power and higher self-esteem as it relates to their intimate partner relationships than they may reveal initially. However, the women are living extremely rough in coping with their intimate partners on a daily basis. Current HIV prevention messages of advising women to avoid sexual relations with partners of unknown HIV status are inherently ineffective (Vogt and Leeper, 2000; Amaro, 1995). These women's ability to get men to comply or even to walk away from noncompliance is complicated by their drug use, financial needs, and unaddressed abandonment issues. Also, just as with other high-risk individuals, women do not disclose their full sexual history at the intake process; therefore, many HIV prevention counselors are performing case management on incomplete or inaccurate sexual histories.

As the women explain, it can be dangerous to educate and empower them without offering their partners the same level of HIV prevention counseling. In fact, this approach to educating and empowering poorer women in our society relative to their male counterparts is similar to the ways in which poor women were provided economic incentives to raise children alone and not have an adult male in the household. History has taught us that this policy resulted in poor family relations and did not save money, as poor children continued to be born into these "undercover family structures" and in fact resulted in poor men having no real place to call home, despite some men's financial and emotional contributions to the family unit.

Women in the Rough want to believe they are capable of being loved and giving love in intimate relationships. Whether women are in denial about their intimate partnership HIV risk factors or whether they reconcile that commitment and condoms in their mind are a contradiction, the fact remains that these women's honest accounts of their intimate partner relationships overwhelmingly reflect a lack of condom use at almost every phase and stage of an intimate relationship. In fact, within paying and casual partner arrangements, condoms symbolize a commodity; but in intimate relationships, they reflect conflict.

In the end, HIV prevention programs designed to address gender and power dynamics must reexamine the strengths and benefits these women gain from intimate relationships. Most of the women have had their children taken away, and many are isolated from their families of origin. This has resulted in these women relying more heavily on the men in their lives to provide emotional, economic, and social support as well as sexual intimacy. So, despite the pain associated with some women's belief that their partners cheat, these women are adamant about trying to be in intimate relationships. Throughout the life course stages of intimate relationships, HIV prevention program coordinators need to understand the emotional connections these women have with their partners despite bouts of frustration, aggression, and violence. In any case, here are some suggestions for HIV prevention programs targeting women at various stages in their intimate relationships.

Stage 1: Courtship. Women who classify their relationships as being in the courtship stage should be encouraged to take an HIV test with their intimate partners as early as possible. As women conclude intimate relationships and begin new courtship processes, they will benefit tremendously from an HIV prevention intervention that helps them to decide to only establish relationships with men who are willing to use condoms from the beginning. As the women highlighted, it is much harder to get men to use condoms after they have had unprotected sex over a period of time in the relationship. Organizations can use a social marketing campaign entitled "Let's Test Together" to promote couples entering new courtship stages to test for HIV prior to engaging in sexual intercourse as the norm for new relationships.

Stage 2: Commitment. Just like mainstream women, the high-risk women in this study desire mutually faithful monogamous sexual relationships with partners known to be uninfected with HIV. HIV prevention counselors can build on this desire as opposed to insisting on safer sex strategies that may conflict with women's intimate relational wishes. Women who are past the initial courtship phase and believe themselves to be in a committed relationship need help in accessing the strengths and challenges of intimate relationships, and how they may be at risk for HIV during the commitment stage of their relationship. In fact, women who had committed partner relationships often asked why the men couldn't come to the counseling. HIV prevention counseling must focus on sessions that strengthen couples' commitment to be in a relationship even if the relationship appears unstable to outsiders. HIV prevention counseling must take into consideration the positive values of intimate sexuality and find a way to build on relationship strengths. Furthermore, HIV prevention counselors must consider whether a couple is trying to procreate, as this serves as a barrier to HIV prevention.

In addition, for women whose committed partners will not attend couples' HIV prevention counseling, I suggest that HIV prevention counselors draw heavily on existing peer stories of women who felt they did not need to protect themselves during the commitment stage, but later tested positive for HIV. The examples must interconnect race, class, and gender standpoints, as high-risk women may not readily identify with cases involving white women or middle-class women.

HIV prevention counselors focusing on building on couples' strengths while addressing their individual and collective risk factors should focus on encouraging committed couples to enroll into drug treatment simultaneously. HIV prevention counselors can build links to drug treatment for couples willing to enter treatment at the same time, but at gender-specific facilities.

Stage 3: Conflict. HIV prevention counselors should focus on helping the women who reveal signs that their intimate relationships are experiencing high levels of conflict understand the heightened risk for HIV during conflict with their partners. One word of caution, however, is that even though women may confide in HIV prevention specialists concerning their intimate partner conflict, many women may not be ready to actually do something different, but rather simply need a sounding board. It may be a more appropriate to inform her on how domestic violence puts women at greater risk for HIV. Specifically, couples in the conflict stage need tools and techniques for better communication; the variety of topics important to couples in general include conflict resolution, financial management, and family relationships. In essence, high-risk couples face similar conflicts as others; however, high-risk couples have fewer resources available for outside mediation and counseling to help them process their differences. At the heart of the suggested guideline for couples in the conflict stage is to offer them aspects of couples' counseling that are available to mainstream couples. An effective module for this phase can be developed in collaboration with local marriage and family counselors.

Stage 4: Compromise. Women who compromise often do so because they believe their choices and options to be limited. HIV prevention programs can help women in the compromise stage address unmet needs, especially for mental health and substance abuse issues. Such an approach may lead to women believing that they have other choices and options. HIV prevention counselors can make referrals for support groups and other options for breaking social isolation. Traditional theories and practices to address gender and power issues in relationships are appropriate for helping women in the compromise stage. It is at this moment that women begin to become more vulnerable to their male partner's risky behavior, as the women compromise their needs and wants in the relationship in order to keep their partner. As HIV prevention case managers discover that women are in the compromise stages of their relationships, they should work with the women to link them to woman-centered institutional support that may raise their consciousness in terms of viable alternatives to remaining in relationships that do not meet their needs.

Stage 5. Conclusion. Clearly, women are the most vulnerable when they attempt to end a relationship, particularly one that is riddled with domestic violence. HIV prevention counselors should work closely with domestic violence guidelines for helping women exit domestic violence relationships. The key, however, is that women must articulate in their own words that they are willing and ready to leave, as it is easy for an HIV prevention case manager to conclude that the women should leave immediately. As much as we would like to see women leave abusive relationships, ultimately it is up to the woman to define herself as being in the concluding stage. It may be more appropriate, however, to present options for concluding high-risk relationships, without making judgmental statements such as "you need to get away from him" or "if you stay, he's going to kill you." Such scare tactics typically have not been enough to convince women to leave and may even shut them down in confiding in the HIV prevention case manager. Thus, presenting strategies and tactics for why and how to conclude harmful relationships in general should be presented as a standard part of HIV prevention counseling for women in intimate relationships in a nonbiased manner.

Finally, as financial support from intimate partners is critically important, women need structural interventions that help them connect to legitimate and stable sources of income (Blankenship, Bray, and Merson, 2000). Clearly, as women exit intimate relationships, they may feel pressured to enter new relationships quickly if it means gaining access to a new source of financial support (Sterk, Elifson, and German, 2000). Specific guidelines and suggestions for addressing women's need for alternative income are addressed in Chapter 6.

Chapter 5

Mothering in the Rough

Most women give up. They give up and they say, take my children.
DFACS take your children or you mama take your children and
they go straight to the street and go straight strung out.

Lisa, a 33-year-old crack cocaine user and mother of three

Given the gaps in knowledge of African-American motherhood in
general, it is no wonder that there are few practical applications for
addressing the needs of high-risk mothers in HIV prevention (Thurer,
1994). The purpose of this chapter on motherhood in relation to HIV
prevention is to present a range of voices and experiences among
high-risk African-American mothers. An analysis of these mothers'
perspectives using black feminist theoretical framework can provide
implications for targeted prevention interventions for African-American
mothers. As the institution of motherhood is central in a discussion of
family systems' impact on HIV risk and resilience, this chapter examines the women's diverse attempts to fulfil the mothering role, despite economic deprivation and addiction. Within the context of HIV
prevention, the concept of motherhood and the roles associated with
mothering are gender-specific issues that have been inadequately
addressed in HIV risk reduction (Dalla, 2004).

The United States' social construction of intensive mothering has
been the source of debate in key American institutions, including family, religion, and the political economy (Hays, 1996). Regardless of
their race or class status, American mothers historically have been expected to make personal changes and sacrifices for their children's

Black Women's Risk for HIV: Rough Living
© 2007 by The Haworth Press, Taylor & Francis Group. All rights reserved.
doi:10.1300/5784_05

well-being, even at the expense of the mother's own mental and physical health. Mothers who do not comply with this good mother role in our society have been subject to punishments that may range in scope of severity (Kearney, Murphy, and Rosenbaum, 1994). Depending on the intersection of a mother's race and class status, as well as her high-risk behaviors, a mother may face criminal punishment for breaking societal norms (Roberts, 1997). This chapter examines the role of mothering as one that impacts a woman's ability and willingness to change her high-risk behavior.

Current literature on motherhood in America provides a clear case for why black feminists must remain committed to writing a discourse on black motherhood being historically distinct from the white counterpart (Collins, 2000). Several authors on motherhood issues highlight the daily dilemmas that mothers face in attempting to balance the conflicting roles of mother and sex worker as socially constructed in American society (Dalla, 2004; Sharpe, 2001; Kearny, Murphy, and Rosenbaum, 1994). In addition, there is a lack of appreciation for the ways in which black women contributed to the upward mobility of middle- and upper-class women throughout history. For example, feminist family researchers argue that during the industrial revolution, affluent white women devoted themselves to raising their families (Hays, 1996), but African-American studies' scholars of that same period argue that it was poor women of color who cared for the children of the affluent (Collins, 2000). Although feminist writers find that intensive mothering in American society began in the early 1900s, they fail to recognize that such emphasis on intensive mothering did not trickle down to poor black mothers—at least not when it came to their own children. Hence, as white mothers were indoctrinated with a culture of intensive mothering, poor women's mothering efforts were commoditized in that they were viewed as the mothers of the future workers for the industrial revolution. Finally, there is little mention in mainstream writings on motherhood of how middle class mothers have historically resolved their intensive mothering dilemma by employing poor black mothers as cheap childcare providers (Collins, 2000; Hays, 1996).

In an effort to fill voids in our knowledge of black motherhood, this study highlights how poor mothers who use drugs cope with contradicting and conflicting roles in our society. While this study focuses on black mothers who use drugs, it is important to note that research (Maher, 1990) profiles the "typical chemical dependent mother as most likely white, divorced or never married, age thirty-one, a high school graduate, on public assistance, the mother of two or three children, and addicted to alcohol and one other drug." However, public discourse generally paints a picture of the typical female addict as "young, poor, black, urban, on welfare, the mother of many children, and addicted to crack." While both types are contradictions in American motherhood, the poor black crack-using mother typically is punished for the harm done to her children, and her white counterpart is treated for her condition (Roberts, 1997).

Over the course of my own fieldwork I was frustrated most by the group of women who were mothers of minor children, especially those who reported having five or more children in the care of various relatives and the foster care system. By the time I studied black feminist thought simultaneously in my gender studies and contemporary theory classes, I pinpointed the source of my frustration. I had felt that this group reinforced the stereotype of black women birthing "crack babies." It did not matter to me that white women were more likely to birth babies craving alcohol; I simply wanted these "crack mothers" to stop embarrassing black mothers by creating the kernel of truth in the crack-baby myth. I found myself often pushing them to go home and spend some time with their children. My study of black feminism helped me realize that I had bought into the controlling images created for black women in general, and crack-using mothers in particular.

Audre Lorde (1996) asserted that, as African-American women who may not be held to a particular controlling image, we must examine "the piece of the oppressor within us." Hence, I bought into the idea that these women made all black women look bad because they continued to have children as crack users. Once I recognized my own short-sighted perspective concerning their present condition, I gave these women the opportunity to define themselves as mothers and to provide meaning of their diverse mothering experiences in the Rough.

In analyzing motherhood as a unique type of family system, I focused on high-risk women's relationships with their minor children. There were two extremes that emerged in explaining the range of perspectives on high-risk women's mothering experiences. On the one hand, women used motherhood as a source of hope and inspiration when they were developing HIV risk management and reduction goals. I refer to this group as "hopeful" mothers. Others I call "hopeless" mothers, as they viewed motherhood from a less hopeful perspective. They found HIV risk reduction goals to be less meaningful because, in their minds, changing would not result in restoring their role and responsibility as primary caregiving mothers.

Hopeful mothers are those who, in general, maintain some level of interaction with their minor children or believe they have an opportunity to become their children's primary caregiver in the future. Four strategies and tactics that are directly linked to hopeful mothers lowering their risk for HIV include: (1) maintaining custody on the margins, (2) giving up temporary custody to kin, (3) disclosing drug use to authorities, and (4) grandmothering as a positive experience.

MAINTAINING CUSTODY ON THE MARGIN

High-risk mothers who maintain custody of their children used several techniques to balance motherhood and high-risk behavior (Hardesty and Black, 1999; Kearney, Murphy, and Rosenbaum, 1994). These mothers are more likely to attempt to smoke crack cocaine in a safer environment and to try to avoid the streets and crack houses in particular. They maintained close ties to extended family members as means of financial and emotional support for their mothering experiences. Even though most do not receive formal child support payments from their children's biological fathers, several mothers have male partners who provide some financial support to help these women care for their minor children.

Mothers who are the primary caretakers for their children under the age of eighteen describe themselves as "heads of household," with living arrangements that include housing projects, housing subsidies, and low market rent for apartments. Primary caregiving mothers are aware of the fact that they have limited financial resources and make attempts to limit crack use when they perceive themselves to be spending money that supports the household. When this is not possible, some women admit that to avoid using household money for drugs, they may occasionally do sex work. In any case, it is important to them to maintain their head of household status and the other benefits often associated with such status (food stamps, Medicaid, and subsidized rent). Therefore, these mothers have a greater incentive to place other priorities ahead of smoking crack, and by doing so they believe they reduce their risk for HIV infection. As Tosha explains, despite balancing competing roles, motherhood remains a high priority in their lives. "I gotta take care of my four children; gotta take care of personal hygiene products for when you done touch me. Then I gotta buy my drugs."

High-risk mothers who maintain custody of their children perceive themselves as having a stake in mainstream society and look down on other mothers as weak and trifling when they lose or give up custody. As hopeful mothers, they attempt to model the caregiving patterns and processes of "normal mothering." Frankie describes her desire to balance normal mothering practices and her crack-using habit.

> My typical day was like getting up, getting my kids ready for school. When they in school, I go and get me a sack or two while they at school. So once I picked them up, I would cook. I go back to being Mama. When they come from school, I'll go back to cooking, cleaning, be done cleaned, whatever. Get them ready and after I did that, I would still go back out and get another one. And that was like my typical day. All of my children always been with me. Regardless of what I done, I'm the one who raised my children. I think that I been bless to still to have a mind, some of my mind, to care for my children and to keep us a place to stay and to send them to school like a normal mother without drugs in her life would be doing. So that's why I judge myself as being a li'l different. But I still have an addiction just as any other crack user.

Lisa describes how she attempts to balance the duties of motherhood and drug use. She also provides a perspective on how mothers who maintain custody seek to distinguish themselves from women who give up on their roles and responsibilities as mothers.

> 'Cause it like this, we [mothers who maintain custody] try to keep us a substantial amount of money. I don't never make my self run completely out of money. I'll try to keep a couple of dollars

here, a couple of dollars there. That's what I mean when I tell you
about my capacity. My mind as a person is still there . . . I don't
let it [crack cocaine] control my whole mind. That why I said
I'm able to maintain my house, pay my rent, keep my children . . .
Most women give up. They give up and they say, take my children. DFACS take your children or you mama take your children and they go straight to the street and go straight strung out.
I ain't with that, 'cause morally I cannot see my children not
being with me after all these years. I done had my oldest son
thirteen years, and I couldn't possibly see my children not being
with me. So even though I smoke, that make me still say, Okay,
what you need? What you need? What you need?

While balancing these roles and responsibilities is a challenge for
mothers in general, it is especially difficult for drug-using women.
Lisa describes how she had been effective in modeling normal mothering behavior, but came face to face with her limitation when her
adolescent son had brain surgery.

He had to go through brain surgery 'cause his brain. They say it
was a birth defect. His brain had overgrowth and got so big that
it growed down into his spine. It was like blocking the blood flow
through his spine. So, fluid set up and it start getting paralysis.
He couldn't feel nothing. And he over my mom. I brought my
other two back home. But since my son got out of the surgery
they trying to give me a Section 8 'cause the lady was saying
that about the conditions of my apartment . . . your son just got
out of brain surgery, you need to get somewhere better . . . It's a
DFACS worker. One of them women that determines whether
you mistreating your children or not and all that.

In this case, the social worker was unaware of Lisa's drug use when
she made a home visit after Lisa's son returned home from having
brain surgery. The social worker arranged for the son to recover at
Lisa's mother's home. Now Lisa is a priority client for getting gov-
ernment-assisted housing. It is unclear how this case would have
evolved had the social worker learned of Lisa's drug use. In other

cases, children have been placed in foster care and mothers ordered to drug treatment.

Like Lisa, Shanté presents a perspective on mothering arrangements in which one daughter lives with her, a son lives with his grandmother, and another daughter is with her father. Shanté's mothering centers on her being able to provide a relatively stable weekday routine while school is in session. On the weekends, however, she sends her daughter to a relative in the suburbs as Shanté's drug selling and use escalates.

> I got three children, but one of them just with me, the other two stay with they daddy. So, I just lug around, take my baby to school. She go to the Boys and Girls Club in the afternoon. She love to participate in everything, especially like talent shows 'cause she like to dance. She said she wanna be a model when she grow up. The children don't have nowhere to play 'round here, so that's why I put mine in the Boys and Girls club, after school. On the weekends I let her over my sister house, 'cause ain't nowhere 'round here for her to play at or nothing like that. 'Cause every corner you turn, somebody standing on the corner selling drugs. The police just riding up and down, so they be shooting and stuff. But down there where I stay, everybody be trying to be like in everybody business at times.

Lois explains how insensitive family members can intervene and say things to the children that undermine even the best attempts to model normal mothering practices. She also provides a glimpse of how children become protective of mothers who are at least trying to fulfill the functions associated with normal mothering.

> I was working at [a] nursing Home. I would take care of my bills, but I always saved me something for my drugs, when that little bit could have went in my house or went on my daughter. I might buy her a few pieces of clothes, but it's money I would take to use drugs with, that's more money that could have went toward her. But she always dressed nice and had nice shoes. Yeah, her aunt told her, your mama up there getting high and this and that. And my daughter would tell them, I got clothes. I got food. I was the type of person that I always took care of bills

and bought her things, but I always snatched me some money back to get high off of.

GIVING UP TEMPORARY CUSTODY TO KIN

Kin as caregivers serve as a source of hopeful mothering by allowing mothers to have a limited role and some responsibilities in their children's lives (Eicher-Catt, 2004). For example, Sabrina, who can only afford a rooming house, does not have adequate housing for her two sons who are in high school. Although her mother has custody of them, Sabrina continues to attend school functions and meetings for her boys, who are in special education programs that encourage parental participation in case review meetings and discipline hearings. Such continued involvement in her boys' lives has resulted in Sabrina setting a new goal of saving money for a two-bedroom apartment, so that her boys can have their own room when spending weekends with her and eventually move in permanently.

> I still stay at a rooming house. And now I got another job. And I been trying to move before this month, because they fixing to remodel the place and they want us to move before April the first. So I'm fixing to find me apartment . . . I had a little problem with my baby boy. He's fifteen. He went to another classroom he wasn't suppose to be in. So the teacher cursed him out, call him stupid retarded child. So he got mad and picked up a stapler and threatened her. Now they kicked him out of school. So we waiting on him to go to court and see when they gonna let him back in. And I talked to the teacher, and said, I'm the same way as my son, but I don't consider myself as retarded and dumb. I said, I gotta a little handicap. He got a little problem. He got a child mind. I said, it wasn't your place to curse him out like that. So, she said she apologized. I said, well since you already took a warrant out on him we had to go through the court.

Women who attempt to balance their drug-using lifestyle and motherhood often find themselves experiencing both role strain and role conflict. Rather than have their children taken from them, they take on a more proactive role of voluntarily giving up custody to kin to avoid interaction with the authorities (Jackson, 1994; Kearney, Murphy, and Rosenbaum, 1994). In comparison to women whose children are forcibly removed by family or social welfare authorities, women who give up custody see this as an act of strength and empowerment. Michelle explains the rationale for why she decided to give up custody of her daughter.

> She was two and I had a one-year-old. So I'm sitting there with two babies in diapers. Still wanted to suck the bottle, both of them. That was running me crazy. So I sent her up there with her cousin 'cause she went up there for the summer. They don't wanna give her back, but I talk to her and I told her, you gone be back down here with Mama don't worry about it. Spoiled to death. She get whatever she wants. They praise her 'cause of her looks. And she got long jet black shiny curly hair. 'Cause when she was born she had a wrap. I mean she taking pictures like this. She spoiled. She get whatever she want. I be talking to her she be like, mommie I'm on the computer.

Women who give up custody view this as a positive choice that could even be framed as risk reduction (Roberts, 1999). In addition, these mothers provide accounts of continued contact in an effort to demonstrate that they remain in touch with children no longer in their custody. They also are quick to point to positive child outcomes and signs of child well-being to validate that they made a good decision in giving up custody. In this way, these mothers find hope in that they sincerely believe in the initial stages that giving up custody is temporary. Janice explains, however, how some children may still be exposed to the drug culture even in kinship care arrangements.

> My dad had got temporary guardianship so welfare and stuff went over to him. My dad was selling drugs and stuff. That was when we was staying on Stewart Ave. I didn't approve of him selling dope around them. 'Cause I'll be laying there sleep and somebody will knock on the door, my son be like, how many? They were little bitty boys one and two-year-olds saying that.

One of the positive consequences of kinship care from the mothers' perspective is it provides an opportunity for making and keeping small promises to their children. Shanese was excited about one such small commitment she was able to make and keep on the day I talked with her. Shanese exclaimed, "I'm going over there [to visit my children] at one thirty. I'm gonna visit. Because my other son, they fixing a li'l dinner for my mom. I wanna be there. My mom's birthday was yesterday and I promised them."

Erica's daughter was removed from her care after being molested at two-and-a-half years old. Because Erica called the police and co-operated with authorities she was able to participate in the decision-making process in terms of identifying kin who were willing to take guardianship of her daughter. Erica prides herself on the fact that every year she celebrates her daughter's birthday at her school with ice cream and cake, and has not missed a year since her daughter started kindergarten and is now eleven years old. Although Erica was able to commit to an annual ritual in the life of her daughter, other mothers struggle to keep promises. For example, Johnsie kept her promise to attend her oldest daughter's high school graduation, but admitted she was only able to stay for fifteen minutes. According to Johnsie, "She graduated in May . . . I probably wasn't there for like fifteen to twenty minutes. I was high, but I was there."

Valerie viewed giving up temporary custody of her newborn to a family member as a hopeful mothering experience. She felt her choice was particularly positive in that the relative was infertile. In addition to keeping the child with kin, she believes she has added value to the family much in the way a surrogate mother might. It is clear from her comments, however, that Valerie is struggling to construct her mothering experience as a positive, given that she is not caring for any of her children.

> I went in labor in the [dope] trap . . . I let my brother and his wife get the baby, 'cause for the simple reason, she can't have no kids. And then my mama got enough as it is. They just got temporary custody. They can't adopt him because the simple reason I'm still living. But as long as it's in the family it's all good. It's bad enough that I don't have the kid, but still I ain't just put him up for adoption and let no anybody get him. Mama wouldn't

split them up. They gone grow up together. Mama said she not gone split them up. So, I think I did the right thing. Well I feel like I did. She can't have no kids and I know he won't be wanting for nothing.

Other mothers commented on how they are able to provide small amounts of financial support for their children. Sharon sets a goal of taking some of her street hustle money to her daughters for school clothes and is able to provide them food stamps that were traded for drugs, although the latter practice is harder to transact in the streets now that the food stamp program takes advantage of electronic bank transfer technology. However, food stamp recipients who are willing to give up their PIN numbers are still able to trade their food stamps for drugs.

> I make sure they have some money and gave them an outfit a week. I still stick to that goal. And when I was really into the game I could send them three hundred to four hundred dollars a piece each weekend and then you know, food stamps. I was able to send books [of food stamps] and send them sixty-five dollar a piece. But then things got rough and I really felt bad 'cause my life so tied up.

Teenagers of mothers who sell drugs in particular may maintain contact with their mothers to get money. However, as Sharon articulates when drug using begins to outweigh drug-selling activities, financial support to children is the first financial commitment to end. Sonya has a teenage son who now is old enough to call and ask for money. Even the day I was talking to Sonya, she commented on how her son had called that very morning from her aunt's house asking her for money for school. Similarly, Allison's adolescent daughter lives in a rural county of Georgia and comes to visit her some weekends when she is in Atlanta with other family members. Allison describes how her mothering experience during these short visits centers on Allison's ability to give her daughter some money.

> [My daughter] still in the country. She been there ever since I went to prison in '87. I had my baby and 'bout six months later, I went to jail. She been with my husband mama ever since.

She come here regular. You'll see her when she come up here.
I hate to see her come in the door. They give her all the money
and stuff when she come. But she come and see her mama and
I still gotta put something in her hand. I'm not gone bring her
here while I'm doing this. My people will kill me if any thang
happen to her. My people will kill me. They would kill me personally and I would deserve to die letting my child go out and
do something. And I'm in a bad neighborhood and she not used
to this.

Allison, like other mothers, rationalized their limited ability to
mother as partly due to the Rough environment, which is not condu-
cive for children to visit even overnight, much less on a daily basis.
Some mothers were adamant that their children were growing up in
neighborhoods where the kids were less aggressive, and that if their
children came to the Rough, they feared they would not be tough
enough to play with the children in this high-risk environment. So, in
their minds, these mothers were actually protecting their children from
danger by not exposing them to the Rough. Doll explains how women
see not bringing their children to the Rough as a positive mothering
tactic.

I moved back over here when I chose to. But I don't like it. The
things that I have seen going on over here, this is not a place to
raise a child. Every corner; each and every corner starting from
Paynes and Kennedy Street all the way 'til you get to Northside
Drive just about. They shooting dope. They smoking dope. It's a
dope trap on every corner.

Johnsie's children are being raised in an affluent suburb of Georgia
with her mother who is a nurse. Johnsie has tried to spend time with
her children; however, they prefer not to come to the Rough.

My kids don't like this area period. My son say the kids over
here are violent. I say, they just regular kids like you . . . He say,
you can't play with them. They take things from them and my
kids ain't used to that. That's not how they was raised.

Hopeful mothers whose children are in kin care often comment on their children's grades, talents, and skills, as well as their future career goals, because part of hopeful mothering is painting a picture of a well-adjusted, normally developing child, with above average looks and grades. This gives them a sense of accomplishment as the birth mother of such children. Moreover, having up-to-date information on their children's most recent report cards, participation in school and community activities, and knowing other unique characteristics about their child's development allows these women to contribute positively to conversations about mothering experiences.

Many women in the Rough have adult children in addition to their minor children. Several of these women's older daughters have taken on the caregiver role for their younger siblings. According to Gloria, "My oldest daughter got my baby. There's no way I'll have her out there like that." This is viewed as a hopeful mothering experience, especially when the older children are integrated into mainstream society, and thus may be able to provide better life chances for their younger siblings. Tosha's four children represent this case well.

> I've been over here thirty years. Got four kids. Got a son in Morehouse. My oldest daughter take care of my two youngest. My son and my daughter take care of the two youngest. She drive them to school everyday. She make sure they got everything they want. She the mama. But she know I did everything I could for them when they were coming up. She just took over. She took them. She didn't have to take them . . . In that welfare reform thing. Eighteen months and you gotta get off. You gotta get a job. I'm a junkie, I can't get no job and keep it. They offered to take my children away from me. My children fine. There's nothing wrong with neither one of my children. My daughter, she just bought a Navigator. Then she got a little house. She got it going on.

Tosha was adamant that she was not on drugs when she raised her first two children. In fact, she started out in the air force after high school and started smoking crack later in life. She believes that her older children care for their siblings in an effort to provide them the kind of drug-free household they grew up in.

DISCLOSING DRUG USE TO AUTHORITIES

Hopeful mothers are not exempt from their interaction with authorities that have the power to remove children from unsafe homes. Hopeful mothers learn over time to be proactive in disclosing their drug use to authorities in hopes that admittance and cooperation will result in leniency or perhaps even assistance in getting into drug treatment. Shanté describes how she disclosed her drug use to emergency room attendants.

> I was pregnant in the tubes 'bout a week ago . . . Friday I just had pain right here on my left side and so I just called the ambulance and they came and told me, I got another one for ya, you pregnant, I say what, Lord have mercy . . . They gave me the ultrasound where they stick something up in ya cervix or something. The man couldn't see nothing in the sack, so he sent me downstairs. The lady found out they was in my left tube. I told them [the emergency room attendants] that I do drugs. They say, you know you shouldn't be doing that. I say yep.

Michelle describes how she used the process of disclosing her drug use to gain access to a safe environment to mother for the first few months after giving birth.

> When I had my son, they didn't test him for nothing. But when the social worker came in there to talk to me and I told her to tell them to test him for drugs, and she said why? I said because I'm a user. So they tested him and I had to go through courts. I was court ordered to go get into a program. I probably would have been worst off than I am now. 'Cause that's what they doing now. Right after you have the baby, they locking you up. And this one girl was telling me she was at the clinic and females was coming in taking pregnancy test, and if their test came back positive, and if narcotics was found in their blood they was getting arrested right there at clinic. So she gone sit up there and tell me to be careful. My doctor know. I let them know my first visit. If tell me if you come back in and your next test positive, then this right here is gone happen, you won't see me no more.

As Michelle explains, she believes she would have been even worse as a mother had she not had a drug-free environment within which to mother in the first few months after giving birth. Michelle and other women confirmed that mothers are threatened by authorities when drugs are found in their system or in that of the baby. While Michelle was fortunate in that she disclosed to a birth attendant who was helpful to her, other women may not be as lucky; many birth attendants make it clear that they are only interested in protecting the child's well-being, even at the expense of the mother's needs (Lieb and Sterk-Elifson, 1995; Roberts, 1991).

GRANDMOTHERING AS A HOPEFUL EXPERIENCE

Like mothering, grandmothering is a gender-specific role and responsibility that has not been adequately incorporated into HIV prevention; there are no HIV prevention programs that specifically target high-risk grandmothers. Women were not only concerned with participating in the lives of their own children; thirteen of them are grandmothers who made additional risk reduction goals of spending time with their grandchildren. According to Pamela, "My biggest regret in life is getting on drugs and missing out on my children and my grandchildren growing up." For Pamela, missing out on the early years of her grandchildren's development was a wake-up call to encourage her to maintain a drug free lifestyle. In fact, several nongrandmothers stated that if they became grandmothers and their children included them in the process of raising their grandchildren, then they would get off drugs. In their estimation, becoming a grandmother on crack has the potential to serve as an incentive for them to begin to show more responsibility. Martha's comment is representative of women who believe that grandmothering would help them lower risk.

> I wish he [her college-educated son] had some kids, 'cause I would ask him to let me get 'em 'cause that would help me do good. Especially a baby. That would help me straighten up. I really would have something to live for, my grandbaby.

Lois confirmed that there may be some validity to Martha's wish for grandchildren as a potential risk reduction motivator. Lois has incorporated nurturing her granddaughter into her daily routine in a way that reduces her participation in high-risk behavior.

> I just pray and keep on going to work and go home and play with my grandbaby and I listen to the tape I got from church and I tell myself I can do it. I don't have no way to get to no NA meetings and then too a lot of times I come home I just want to take a shower, cook, and lay down.

Similarly, Sunnie, who has eight grandchildren, discussed the importance of grandmothering as a risk reduction technique. Currently, she spends time with her newest grandchild and has less time to be in the street and smoking crack.

> They just encouraged me to find other things to occupy my mind. I have eight grandchildren so I started spending time with them. And every little money that I get go to the baby. You know that's important to me. I didn't get a chance to do this for her little boy but this little girl I'm doin' better. Well, mostly the baby comes up and I don't have time for streets. Having that baby helps me. She [the HIV prevention counselor] just put an impact on my life.

Sunnie is now involved in helping her daughter remain clean as a requirement for keeping her newborn baby. She attends Narcotics Anonymous meetings with her and is happy to be a part of this grandchild's life, because she described having been too high to be a support to her children and her first seven grandchildren. According to Sunnie, she uses the newborn baby as a reason to stay out of the streets. Not only is she involved in her grandchildren's lives, but she also supports her daughter in her recovery. She proudly announced, "I go to meetings with Kayla, and I enjoy it. That's the reason I'm halfway out here."

HOPELESS MOTHERS THEMES

The women categorized as hopeless mothers portrayed a plethora of emotions, including signs of clinical depression, anger, and rejection. Most were pessimistic about their chances of "normal motherhood." Various aspects of hopeless mothering were shared in four main themes: (1) no contact with children, (2) death of a child, (3) negative interactions with authorities, and (4) teen daughters becoming pregnant.

Hopeless Mothering

Hopeless mothering in general refers to mothers who perceive themselves as not being able to care for their children in an effective manner. In addition, hopeless mothering is highly associated with stress and guilt among high-risk women, as they believe their chances of functioning as normal mothers are limited. Hopeless mothers also describe themselves as being in a vicious cycle of being stressed, because they are unable to mother and use high-risk behavior as a way to cope with the pain. Over time, however, high-risk behavior takes more time and money—two key resources needed to care for children—thus leaving the mother even further alienated from using steps toward effective mothering as an HIV risk reduction strategy.

Portia provides a perspective on how high-risk women may arrive at a state of hopeless mothering and how such thinking is interconnected to her unwillingness to attempt to lower her risk for HIV prevention. I asked Portia if she had changed her sexual behavior as part of the intervention process and she replied, "No! For what? I ain't changing. I'm just going to be me. I don't care. Do or die 'cause my kids aren't with me." Portia believes that she had no reason to make changes because it would not result in her getting her family back. Several crack-using mothers are bombarded with messages from family members and social service providers that they should make changes in their lives in order to get their children back or to take better care of them. Portia's mother now has full custody of her three children and has taken them to a southwestern state. According to Portia, after years of attempting to help, her mother finally severed ties completely between Portia and the children. Now, Portia has a difficult time finding anything worth making changes for in life. So Portia, like other crack-using mothers, has come to internalize steps toward changed behavior as being not for themselves, but for their children's best interest.

Men in general are seldom confronted with the idea of making changes in their lives in order to be better caretakers. Moreover, men who do drugs seldom face the added pressure of getting clean for any-one's well-being except their own. In comparison, women are stigmatized and made to feel that their changed behavior should not be for themselves. Such stigma and selfishness are linked to the ideology of patriarchy and serve as a justification for the devaluation of women in general. In the case of the creation and implementation of drug rehabilitation along masculine values, inequality is subtle in that on its face, these facilities appear gender neutral. However, the fact that drug rehabilitation centers have not transformed to meet the needs of women crack users highlights the hegemonic perspective that "good girls" don't do drugs in the first place.

Poor African-American women fight an even stronger controlling image of child caretaker from an historical perspective. Not only are they as drug users unable to care for their own children, but they cannot care for other people's children, which has been their assigned role in America since slavery. As Collins (1991b) articulates, when white women entered the labor market in the post–World War II era, they challenged white patriarchal power. However, white women's liberation often meant poor black women's further subordination as the latter fulfilled the housekeeping and childcare duties of their white counterparts.

I asked Portia what she wanted in the future. She asserted that in a year from the time I talked to her she wanted to be drug free. In addition, she responded, "I want a husband. I want a family. I want it to be right. And money, and the damn picket fence. That's what I want." I remember thinking, "That's what I want too." I felt I had made a connection with her and proceeded to ask if she felt she could make changes. Without hesitation, she stated, "I've learned to say no to 'Juicy Fruit' [her ex-boyfriend]. I feel I can make a bunch of changes. But until I see something better that I can accomplish, then I can really do something for myself."

For Portia, long-term changes need to be tied to seeing herself accomplish something associated with mainstream life. After an initial goal of wanting to be drug free, the rest of Portia's goals could have been a quote from almost any middle-class American mother. In fact, before drugs, Portia lived in a solid middle-class neighborhood where she witnessed families living the American dream. Perhaps her decision not to make changes is tied to her perception that the be-

havioral changes taught at the HIP House would only help her remain
HIV negative, but would not promise a return to her middle class
status and motherhood.

Doll acknowledges that she walked away from a "controlling" relationship in which she balanced mainstream roles of housewife, business partner, and mother to three small children. As Doll increased
her participation in high-risk behavior, she recognized that she spent
less and less time with her children. Doll recently began prostituting
herself and living in a rooming house, where sex and drugs are a
part of everyday life. She perceives herself as being unable to make
changes because her three children are not part of her life. Currently,
they are living with their father, and Doll feels that she is "deep down
in a circle where there is no way of getting out . . . because my children not with me."

Women described the process of hopeless motherhood as one that
perpetuates misery. The more they think about the harm they perceive
themselves to be causing their children, the more miserable they become concerning their self-worth within the context of motherhood.
According to several women, this misery leads to increasing risky behavior to mask the pain, which removes them further from the role of
"normal" mother in their children's lives.

No Contact with Children

Mothers distinguished between feelings associated with not having
custody and not having contact with children. Mothers who do not
have custody, but still have contact—even if they choose not to interact—believe they have some hope in developing a relationship with
their children. On the other hand, mothers who have no contact with
their children perceived this as a barrier to their willingness and ability to focus on HIV prevention. Women discussed several conditions
under which they may lose contact with their children, ranging from
being barred by family members to being officially barred from the
child when the nonkin foster care arrangements are ordered.

> My li'l girl stay with her daddy in Griffin. My li'l girl birthday
> was yesterday. He wouldn't let me see her. And my li'l boy he's
> in DFACS. So I'm trying to get him back. He was here with me
> and he was down this lady house and I used to have him sleep

somewhere 'til I be decent. I was on the street but I know I don't
want to have my son like that. And I went there and he had left
and went with his friends downtown and got caught stealing.
But he never wanted for nothing. I don't care how many drugs
I did, I gave my baby. He just doing what other child do, that's
all. I just want my children back.

For a variety of reasons the family caretaker may decide to prevent
the mother from seeing her children. When caregiving relatives cut
off contact, mothers view this as a state of hopelessness in relation to
their ability to make changes in other areas of their lives. Generally,
this happens when the mother upsets the children or makes promises
she is unable to keep. In any case, if the mother was allowed to visit
her children in kinship care, she could also use this time to cool out
from drugs and other high-risk behaviors. So, not only does losing
contact equate the mother with not having an opportunity to interact
with her children, but now she will need to find an alternative place to
"cool out" or take a break from drug use. When mothers do not have
access to these familial homes for cooling out, they typically resort to
high-risk environments and behavior.

Some mothers felt hopeless in breaking a cycle of abandonment
that their own mothers had demonstrated in their mothering experiences. Jennifer is frustrated with herself, as she believes that she is
modeling the behavior of her own mother. Jennifer, who spent most of
her young life in and out of foster care, explains how she feels. "My
kids stay with my aunt. My oldest son, his daddy. It's all kind of punishment. 'Cause I'm gonna get my son back. I feel like I'm doing the
same thing my mama carried us through. I'm so mad and pissed off at
myself." Although her children are in kinship care and not with
strangers as she was, she is able to make the connection that she has a
lot in common with her own mother's ineffective mothering behavior.

Janice describes the process of losing hope as she lost contact with
her child. Her story shows how the family members may be doing what
they believe is in the best interest of the child without considering the
mother's feelings and ability to mother at some level.

My nine-year-old, my daughter, she with her dad. She been with
her dad since she was eight months. And my seven-year-old,
I ain't seen him since he was two years old. The first time we

had sex the rubber burst and I got pregnant with him. So we moved together and it was his first child. He was religious. I'm smoking and all that . . . We goes to Alabama one weekend, my baby was six months, so they was like, Janice, let li'l Bo stay down here for awhile to you get yourself together . . . Every time he got ready to go to Alabama, he'll come see me for sex. He'll pay me for sex and stuff or just ride by and see me. Then he'll say, I'm going to Alabama. Everything went on. Then, he'll say, Bo coming up the weekend. You want me to come get you? So when his family from Alabama come to Atlanta they go to the aunt's house. So he'll say, Jr. coming to Atlanta on the weekend, he gone be over Sally house. I go to see him and they go into the third degree. This happened up until he got two years old. He seven now. I ain't seen or heard a trace on him. His aunt number still the same. I call her and she say he been lying and saying he was bringing my son to see me. It been five years and I ain't seen him in five years. She say she couldn't even believe it. She ain't gone tell me nothing 'cause they family. She say he bring my son over there. I can't never catch them, but she say, I'll get him the weekend so you can see him. But when she say that and I'll call, it don't go through.

The Death of a Child

When a mother who uses drugs experiences the death of a child, she is highly likely to smoke more drugs as a coping mechanism. The women in this study described the pain associated with a child's death. There were some mothers whose children died as young babies, and others whose children were killed, typically as teenage boys involved in drug-selling activities. While mothers experiencing both kinds of death grieve, the issues are different. On the one hand, mothers whose children die when they are still young babies find a sense of peace in that the child will not have to experience the high-risk environment nor face the trajectory of drama and trauma that many children of poor drug-using mothers experience in trying to mother effectively. Pamela explains how mothers process the loss of children who died at birth.

I got three [children] living. And one dead. She would be ten. She was stillborn . . . A combination of [drugs] and then the night before I went into labor, me and my first husband got into it and he threw me down a flight of stairs. So, all that contributed, plus my drug usage. It was a blessing 'cause when they did the autopsy, they said had she lived she would have been a vegetable. So it was best that she go on. I can deal with that better than have had her here and then she died. I mean I went through my own grieving process. As a matter of fact her birthday was the twenty-third of this month. She would have been eleven. I'm going through my own little thing right now. I got this little prayer I say . . . Lord give me strength and guidance to get through it. And there was something that kept saying, go get you fix; go get you a fix. Get a crack rock. That will help soothe it on over. The day will be over soon. I kept saying, oh no!

Frankie's son was killed in a drug-related incident. She describes how this tragedy resulted in her smoking more drugs.

My oldest son would have been twenty but he got killed. He was one of those that wasn't out there. I'm not defending him. I'm not trying to make him look good or whatever because he wasn't. He was, like . . . in the tenth grade going to the eleventh grade. He left out the house. He was smoking a blunt and they was mad 'cause he wouldn't let them hit it that Friday. They tried to treat him like he was just a li'l boy. And that day, it was broad daylight, and they told me to come and get my child; he had been shot. And when that happened, that really did my world. Girl, I started smoking too. And like, right today, no excuse, but I would rather smoke than to think about what I dealt with and what I have to deal with. I do 'cause it hurts. It's terrible, girl. It's hard. It's hard. It's hard. And I deal with it right today. I deal with it. The worst thing for me to deal with is to think about it. Girl, I be sleep sometime and I can't go to sleep. I be laying there and it be getting in my mind so hard 'bout the look he gave me when he was on the ground and the thought of the pain going through his body and me being his Mama, you know. Just thinking about when he hit the ground. All of that! That stuff terrible! That's hard. I never thought about burying one of my children, but when I buried my baby, that messed my mind up. That messed my life up. That messed me up.

While Frankie's son was killed some years prior to her HIV prevention intervention, Lolita's son was recently killed, which served as the primary reason why she wanted to enter the HIV prevention program as a way to gain access to a counselor. She explains how she heard an outreach worker describing the program and thought it may help to talk to someone about her problems.

> I heard [the outreach worker] talkin' about it. He was tellin' someone else about it. And I told him I was so depressed. I had just lost my son and I was so depressed. And everybody that you talk—when you say something to them they don't understand your feeling. You get to say it but they want you to hear what they got to say . . . When I came in here I felt so relieved. 'Cause it was so much pressure off of my mind. His supposed-to-be friends had him set up. He was sellin' dope. And believe me when they called me and told me my baby was dead! I still love him. Sometimes I still think my mind play tricks on me.

Lois sums up the need for helping mothers cope with the loss of a child as part of HIV prevention. She further suggests that helping mothers cope with loss needs to be a core program component that primarily relies on peer supporters to help women through the grieving process and not use this period as a time to self-medicate with drugs.

> I mean how can tell me something if you have never been there. Like I have had some kids to die. People say, I know how you feel. You haven't had your kids die or got killed, you don't know that feeling, so you can't say.

Negative Interactions with Authorities

For mothers who use crack cocaine, negative interaction with authorities often begins during prenatal care. Some women self-select prenatal care; however, many do so later in their pregnancy and miss some vital care specifically geared to strengthen fetus development in the first trimester. Others are court ordered to prenatal care to protect the unborn child from the harmful effect of drugs. Although Johnsie self-selected prenatal care, her story provides a perspective on why women who use drugs may seek to avoid prenatal care.

He was lucky. He was an angel. I call him an angel because I smoked a lot of crack and a lot of cigarettes and did a lot of dranking because his father, we don't even get along . . . can't stand him. He don't like me and I don't like him. I was doing a lot of stuff. At first I was really trying to abort that baby, but God say no, no, no, you goin' to have this one. This going to be your lesson to learn right here. He weighed nine pounds. They told me that if I come back into Grady Hospital to have another crack baby they was going to lock me up. They told me that when I was getting prenatal care and every time they drawed blood I was zooted up. They say, you keep coming in here with drugs in your system and you know you pregnant. I say, I'm gonna stop, I'm gonna stop. Soon as I left that hospital from prenatal care, I was toot, toot! [She shows me how she lights up]. I know I was wrong.

As Johnsie describes, prenatal care providers' negative interactions and even verbal threats toward pregnant addicts can result in these women taking their chances on the streets and foregoing prenatal care in a way that could be more harmful for both mother and child. Even women who are brave enough to face the reprimands of prenatal care providers still find themselves stressed and using drugs while pregnant. In fact, just as Johnsie alluded to, at least two other women in the study confided that in an effort to avoid potential criminal punishment for doing drugs while pregnant, they deliberately tried to miscarry their unborn child. Tosha, however, stood tough in facing the authorities after her baby was born.

I told them if they stuck my baby one more time I was going to sue them. 'Cause my baby didn't have no drugs in her system. It's all because I get on my knees and pray that's why. God made a way. I asked God not to do that to my baby. Don't take it out on my baby 'cause of what I do.

Mothers who experience negative interactions with child welfare personnel generally describe themselves as hopeless mothers. This is especially the case when children are taken within the first year of birth. This is the case with Mona.

My children in foster care. I don't see my children. My little girl is in foster care and my son is in prison for robbery and riding in stolen automobile. [My daughter] been in foster care since she three or four months old. She be ten, June sixth . . . I been foster child all my life 'cause my mama and my daddy used to mistreat. I got out of foster care and I came down here. I just got put out of my apartment day before. My stuff sitting out in the street. I had to sell some of my stuff from off the sidewalk. Had a little bit of money in my pocket. I hate to be selfish. I didn't want to be taking her back and forth to no shelters. So, I let another lady take my baby. I didn't want her out in the street. She had two daughters who took care of the baby while she at work. And the hospital called and said my baby been dropped. I get down to the hospital. I'm drunk. She went and took my baby and I ain't never seen my baby no more. I'm trying to get myself together 'cause when [my son] seen me last time I look like a rag doll rubbed in shit. I do be ashamed. I do. I be ashamed when I do like 'is.

Punkin's son was taken into foster care while she was incarcerated and also tested positive for HIV.

I was incarcerated. I was pregnant with Malcolm, and they told me. But I didn't believe it 'cause he didn't come out with it. They took them when I was in State Prison. State took them when he was three days old. 'Cause I was incarcerated.

As I observed Mona and Punkin, I couldn't help but make some connections between their past and present lives within the context of the negative interactions they experienced with authorities concerning their own children. First, both Mona and Punkin grew up in foster care and began prostituting at an early age. In addition, both were diagnosed as clinically depressed and have chosen to avoid mental health services. Even though they are twenty years apart in age, both have experienced domestic violence and limited attachment to the job market. Clearly, there is a need for further research to understand how girls in foster care are at heightened risk for HIV infection.

Teen Daughters Becoming Pregnant

Earlier I discussed how women described the grandmothering experience as an element of hopeful mothering. In contrast, the process of learning that one's teen daughter is pregnant is initially perceived as a hopeless mothering narrative. Most women described how the latter learned to accept and embrace their teen daughter's pregnancy after initially experiencing a range of emotions ranging from sadness to outrage. Despite their own high-risk behavior, these mothers reject the discourse that they are indifferent to or even supportive of their teen daughters' involvement in sex. These mothers did not want their teen daughters to end up as unmarried mothers and potential high school dropouts with limited education and economic earning potential. Although they recognize their daughters are more likely to become teen mothers in the first place, these mothers are still upset when they learn of their teen daughters' dilemma. Drug-using mothers are not only upset that their daughters are pregnant teens, but also because they are unable to support their daughters through this period. Sharon was a teen mother and knows what her own daughter must be experiencing in some aspects.

> She has a baby. And it's like I wasn't there for her. None of her pregnancy. And like right now that's eating me up. But, it's like her and my auntie start falling out. I'm gonna cry. And when she started falling out up there. I was staying with this and that and I couldn't even tell her to come home. Well wherever I was, I would have made it home but it wasn't right with the way she was living. I didn't want her to see how I could fall into this trap.

Lois has maintained custody of her three children throughout her drug use largely due to the financial and emotional support provided by her non–drug-using husband. However, she described feeling like a failure when her 15-year-old daughter became pregnant.

> I was mad; I was hurt; I asked her, I say, Tiffany, have you had your period. Yeah; I'm sturdy checking the trash can. I ain't seen no pads. I say, Tiffany, I'm going to tell you like this 'cause you know I'm crazy. Is it a possibility that you pregnant 'cause I'm taking you to the doctor on Monday. She say, yeah. I'm thinking the baby going to come in December or January right. I take her to the doctor, they holler June. I could see my grand-baby just as good on the ultrasound. I say, this baby is developed. She had that baby in May. I took her in April. I was there when she had it. She went in labor that night. The whole house was

drunk. I had smoked some dope. I say, you would have to wait until we do all this. I went in there and brush my teeth, washed my face, and changed my clothes. I ain't want to go down there smelling. She asked for an epidermal. I say, no. She say, Mama why? I say, No, I want you to remember these pains so you won't come back down here having another baby at an early age. So about an hour before the baby came I let them give her one. I seen my grandbaby come out. I cut the umbilical cord. They were going to lay the baby on her chest. She say no, please don't, that baby so nasty. Don't touch me. I say, but that's your baby. She say, I don't care, that baby nasty. So they washed the baby off. They give them something for hepatitis or something; they gave her first shot. She looked at the baby and she looked at me. She say, I messed up, didn't I? I say, you sure did. You lost your freedom. [Her baby daddy] in jail now. He was out then. When I left there, I came home to bath and cook to take her dinner back. I seen this little black, skinny, red-eye guy in there. I say, who is this? Everybody looked at me. So I get real crazy and loud. Somebody going tell me something about who he is. So my sister-in-law say, that's Don, that's my cousin. I say, so why he down here? She say, that's my baby daddy.

CYCLING BETWEEN HOPELESS AND HOPEFUL MOTHERING

Kawana's Case

This section highlights two case studies of how women cycle through bouts of hopeful and hopeless mothering across the life course. I draw heavily on the analytic and theoretical framework used by O'Leary and Martin (2000), as they used the case study approach to examine one woman's risk factors across the life course. In this case, I am using mothering experiences across stages that highlight missed opportunities to intervene appropriately in the lives of mothers at risk for HIV infection. For example, Kawana's mothering experience can be analyzed in eight distinct stages that result in fluctuations between hopeful and hopeless mothering (Table 5.1).

TABLE 5.1. Conditions of hopeful and hopeless mothering.

Stage 1 Hopeless mothering	Stage 2 Hopeful mothering	Stage 3 Hopeless mothering	Stage 4 Hopeful mothering	Stage 5 Hopeless mothering	Stage 6 Hopeless mothering	Stage 7 Hopeful mothering	Stage 8 Hopeful mothering
Becomes pregnant as a crack user	Gives birth and gains access to welfare, food stamps, and Medicaid	Fails at balancing the roles of mother and crack user	Places child in temporary custody of kin while she attempts to go into drug treatment	Leaves drug treatment and goes back to life of drug use and sex work	Kin's temporary custody of child lapses into full custody	Enters HIV prevention program (ten years later) and sets goals to get drug free and begin interaction with son	Gets clean; becomes gainfully employed with a living wage job; begins weekend day visits; begins paying child support

Kawana's aunt took temporary custody of her 2-month-old son while she went into a drug treatment program. However, Kawana left the program within a week because she could not identify with the approach and the other people in the program. Nor did she make a connection with the white male psychiatrist. According to Kawana, the facility was a psychiatric hospital located in an upper middle-class community servicing primarily white males addicted to cocaine. She described having "Ritz Carlton"-type hospitality, but made no connection with this group of addicts in terms of her experiences in the Rough as a female crack user and sex worker. After a thorough psychiatric exam the doctor released her and she returned to the only home she knew in the Rough. Soon hopeful mothering gave way to hopeless mothering as her aunt's temporary custody lapsed into full custody. Over time, her interaction with her son was limited due in part to her own obsession with drug use, but also due to her aunt's rules of limited contact with her son, stating that he acted out whenever Kawana visited and left. Kawana now has returned to a state of hopeful mothering as she has been clean for five years, kept a steady living wage–paying job, and maintained a two-bedroom apartment. Although her son only visits on the weekend, she has, even with this level of interaction, increased her hope and determination to remain drug free and HIV negative.

Kawana's narrative represents how women can transition from hopeful to hopeless fairly quickly. While her interaction with the social worker appeared positive, her encounter with the drug counselor left her hopeless in terms of getting off crack cocaine as a first step in regaining custody. According to Kawana, she had been prostituting herself without protection for a year prior to getting pregnant. She admits that she expected the doctor to tell her that she and her child were HIV positive. Finding out they were both negative, however, led to her attempting to play the role of mother, which propelled her back to a state of hopeful mothering.

> The first six months after having my li'l boy I had food stamps and welfare. He stayed with me then. I was trying to stay off dope. I was still doing it and it was bothering me. I didn't want family children services to come there and take him from me. They say when children born with crack in they system they

come and do random visits. I would run out the door while he was sleep and time it because babies have them four-hour schedules. And sometimes I would come back in he done woke up and crying. I'm geeked and trying to hold him. I was feeling like he knew something was different 'cause he wouldn't stop crying. And that just would bother me. I talked to my caseworker and I told her that I wanted to go into treatment. I wanted my aunt to get temporary custody of him while I was in there. I went to a hospital out in [a suburban community]. It wasn't no crack addicts out there. It was cocaine heads. I was the youngest person. They told me they didn't have a crack program. They were getting treated for anxiety and mental things. It wasn't what I thought. It was set up like I was in the Ritz Carlton. You in a room by yourself, and you ring the buzzer. I stayed about a week but it wasn't anything they could do for me there. The doctor evaluated me and said it wasn't a reason for me to stay. So when I got out of there I just went back. I kept saying I was going to get into another program and temporary custody lapsed into full custody. So, he's been there every since.

Despite her own actions to reduce risk, Kawana interpreted the psychiatrist's message to mean that there was no help for people on crack cocaine at that time and at that facility. Such feelings of helplessness led to her eventually returning to the streets and reengaging in high-risk behavior for the next nine years. When she decided to try rehabilitation again in a program consisting primarily of other crack users, her motive remained that of wanting to clean up for an improved relationship with her now ten-year-old son. Like other mothers, Kawana recognizes that regaining full custody may not be in the best interest of the child, but because her son remained in the family, she would like to be in a better position to participate in his childhood.

Pamela's Case

There are some mothers who use drugs and still manage to bond with their children and have a history of caring for and nurturing them. When their children are taken away, they can find a source of strength that may be different from that of mothers like Kawana, who gave up temporary custody in the first few months after giving birth.

For example, Pamela's ten-year-old son had always been in her care, despite her heroin and crack cocaine habits. However, Pamela tearfully described her interaction with a social worker as she was facing a child neglect charge when authorities were contacted either by the school or a neighbor. Pamela is still unsure of how they found out her son may not have been properly being cared for.

> When they came in I was using and then they found out I was about to lose my house and somebody had tipped them off. So the same social worker I had been working with came by and at that time it was a false alarm 'cause I had it going on. And then she came the other time and it was justified 'cause I had just finished getting high. She said, Pamela I can just look at you. The first time she came, she took and tore the paper up, but this time when she didn't take and tear that paper up I knew it. She took my son outside and then the police pulled up outside. I knew then they was getting ready to take him. So they took him outside and put him in the police car and talked to him. Then they came back about five minutes later and went and got his clothes . . . She said we got to take him because you are unfit and you can get him back when you get some help. They said they could take my full parental rights away because, see, a lot of them have had their full rights taken and they put them up for adoption. But she told me I can get mine back because she knows what type of person I was. And she was so proud of me now. She gave me a certificate when we were in court last week . . . last Tuesday. The same day I told them to cut the plug on my dad. It was joy and it was sadness. But the joy overturned the sadness. I said, my dad is in a better place. He's out of his misery. 'Cause he was just brain damaged anyway. I left there and then I went to court. And they said, how are you standing this? I said, I got a good God, the God of my chosen. I'm grieving in my own way. I'm still grieving. But, they say, you been doing good. Yeah, I have to go every two weeks to get tested. I go over there to Boulevard in the outpatient. And they faxed them my results and told them I been attending the meetings and everything. They said they know I don't have the proper housing right now, but they went ahead and said they going to overlook that 'cause I been doing every-

thing so good. I told them I am still affiliated with you all and everything was just positive. And then my caseworker gave me a certificate of congratulations on getting my child back.

As a mother, Pamela perceived her interaction with the social workers, drug counselors, and other authorities to be positive because she believed in her ability to complete the necessary action steps for regaining custody. Such hopefulness and subsequent activity in antic- ipation of reuniting with her son ultimately resulted in reducing her risk for HIV infection.

PRINCIPLES TO GUIDE ADDRESSING ISSUES RELATED TO MOTHERHOOD AS HIV PREVENTION INITIATIVES

In keeping with a black feminist perspective, the principles pre- sented in this section serve as guidelines for enhancing existing HIV prevention interventions for more relevance in the lives of mothers. Specifically, in keeping with a black feminist perspective, the guide- lines are discussed within the context of structure and agency per- spectives and have implications for more effective HIV interventions targeting poor African-American mothers who smoke crack cocaine.

The first generation of HIV prevention models were less concerned with motherhood as a barrier or facilitator to one's ability to reduce the risk for HIV (Archie-Booker, Cervero, and Langone, 1999). While gender and power theory have provided a framework for ad- dressing gender-specific HIV prevention issues, black feminist theo- retical perspectives are more appropriate in understanding black women and their risk for HIV. As indicated throughout this chapter, women's own narratives about their mothering experiences can guide new HIV prevention programs targeting high-risk mothers. Dynamics such as daily living conditions and circumstances as well as resources that high-risk mothers have at their disposal impact mothers' ability and willingness to focus on HIV prevention. Closely related to that for mothers who have lost custody of their minor children is the need to understand how long the mother cared for the children prior to their separation, who took custody, how long the children have been out of the mother's care, and the degree to which mothers currently interact with their children. What we know less about, however, is what family caregivers in particular tell children of high-risk mothers about their parent's condition and how this may impact the mother's continued risk for HIV (Battle et al., 1996).

Culturally relevant HIV prevention programs can help service providers understand how historically distorted images of poor black mothering experiences may impact these women's choices today in ways that place them at risk for HIV infection. Service providers also can benefit from learning about the historical strengths and challenges associated with black motherhood in America. As the women's narratives confirm, they avoid prenatal care and hospital deliveries because of the real and perceived maltreatment they may encounter from authorities. However, if these places became a safe place for both mother and child, these women may be able to receive effective risk reduction. In essence, structural changes must take place in the thinking and practices among maternal and child health institutions that support a shift from criminalizing their pregnancies to medicalizing them.

There is a need for cultural and gender sensitivity training among diverse groups of service providers who may come into contact with mothers who use drugs. The primary learning objective needs to focus on helping social service staff representing various agencies address their own biases and prejudices toward mothers who use drugs. Simply put, there is a tremendous need to teach and coach service providers on how to assist women coping with a wide range of mothering circumstances. Closely related to that is the need to educate service providers toward helping clients locate motherhood mentally and physically along a continuum of hopeful and hopeless mothering experiences.

HIV prevention program developers should focus on specific modules that can be used as an additional prevention case management session for mothers. In particular, modules should be developed that distinguish between reducing risks among mothers whose children are still in their care, as well as among mothers who have some contact and even no contact with their children. In addition, there is a need for some suggested activities and interactions that help mothers engage emotionally in their children's lives with minimum disruption in the child's everyday routine. At the same time, we need to communicate to social service providers that, for various reasons, some women are not interested in regaining custody or interacting with their children.

Chapter 6

When Work and Welfare
Disappear in the Rough

The Rough ain't full of nothing but hustle!

Stephanie, a 43-year-old heroin user

This chapter is grounded in the black feminist theme of "unique experiences" among African-American women attempting to earn money after work and welfare have disappeared in Rough-like environments. Clearly the disappearance of work and welfare has implications for women's HIV risk and protective factors. For example, as work disappeared among men, the clientele for sex work changed over time. Women asserted that sex work is very much a part of trickle-down economics in that when there is a recession in general or massive job loss in sectors dominated by males, the demand for sex work is diminished. Women discussed how men who, in the past, had spent hundreds of dollars partying with sex workers, curtailed or eliminated this activity altogether over the last four years during our country's economic downturn. In addition to joblessness, welfare reform also resulted in a new group of women taking to the streets to perform sex as a survival strategy. Moreover, men who have sex with men have emerged as additional competition among female sex workers. This oversupply of sex workers makes the Rough a buyers' market for the most part, with Johns being able to demand what they want at reduced prices. Thus, the impact of joblessness in the inner city and welfare reform has resulted in a change of terms and players in the sex trade. This change has led to women in the Rough becoming more creative in how they make a living in the Rough. This chapter specifically highlights how such strategies and tactics to earn money can serve as HIV risk and protective factors.

The inspiration and insight to examine the ways in which women in the Rough make a living beyond selling drugs and sex is grounded in my own recollection of hustles in my old poverty-stricken neighborhood, in which most households had insufficient funds to make ends meet. I recall my own grandmother collecting old clothes all year long to hand make quilts and sell them for fifteen to twenty-five dollars to supplement her SSI monthly check and food stamps. My mother provided transportation for working-class men and women in the neighborhood to the bus stop or work sites between 5:30 a.m. and 6:00 a.m. She also provided rides for women on the weekends to the grocery store and Laundromat for extra money. Other women in the neighborhood supplemented their welfare checks and food stamp allowances by making prom dresses and homecoming gowns. Also, we had a term for hairdressers in our neighborhood called "kitchen-ticians," meaning women and girls who styled hair in their homes as opposed to a beauty salon. In fact, this was my younger sister's hustle; as early as thirteen years old, she was talented in cutting and coloring hair in the latest styles. My own hustle stemmed from a skill I developed while living with my grandmother in the first thirteen years of my life, when I learned to sew. Even without a sewing machine I made money hemming pants and starching jeans to a crisp.

I vividly remember bake sales of homemade pound cakes, red velvet cakes, and chocolate cupcakes sold by various women in the neighborhood for extra money. We had candy ladies and ice cream houses where we could stretch a dollar for after-school snacks. Other women operated full-fledged soul food restaurants right out of their government projects to provide meals to working families, allowing them to pay in food stamps. Working men bought lunches to take to suburban construction work sites when they could find work. I also remember these same women feeding children in the neighborhood whose parents neglected them, instead of involving child protective services. So the idea that the women in this study would have skills and knowledge to hustle as a way of supplementing their income grew out of my own unique experiences of watching African-American women strategize on how to survive despite socioeconomic and social policy limitations.

In addition to the positive aspects associated with women seeking to lower their risk for HIV as they participate in diverse moneymaking ventures, I highlight how these women's moneymaking strategies can be viewed as exploitation by dominant groups who benefit from these women's cheap labor power in the Rough. As these women remain part of a growing underclass relegated to serve in the army of cheap labor, it is important to understand how there may be limited incentives among mainstream stakeholders to provide these women with better economic options. In essence, even if they cleaned up from drugs, most would only be eligible for jobs that pay at lower than living wages, lack health care benefits, and have harsh working conditions (Edin and Lein, 1997). In like manner, these women are exploited by mainstream and middle-class drug users, using them to gain access to drugs without risking their own personal safety in the Rough.

In examining how women cope financially in the aftermath of work and welfare disappearing, I wanted to understand the complexity of compounded issues among the women in this study as it relates to employability in general, including criminal records, chronic drug abuse problems, limited job skills, and spotty ties to the mainstream workforce, as well as a lack of references or permanent contact information. In an effort to understand how women cope with economic and employment limitations, I asked, "What are women doing to make money in the Rough?" The typical answer to this question was "turning dates." However, when I asked women to explain their unique approach to making money, many had some other hustle as a first choice, and turning dates was the last resort. I began to inquire about "what other hustles are going on out there" as a way to get specific strategies and tactics that women were using to make money other than sex work and selling drugs. This resulted in several themes of "hustling" including "hustling knowledge," which is divided into two subthemes: hustling one's knowledge of drugs in the Rough and hustling one's knowledge of sex in the Rough.

HUSTLING KNOWLEDGE

The concept I use to describe the process of hustling knowledge is that of "going between for the mainstream." For many women, hustling knowledge of the sex trade and drug availability in the Rough has become a viable alternative to actually performing sex work or selling drugs themselves. To be sure, this means that women are constantly observing other women to determine who is desperate enough to perform high-risk sex in ways that women in the study could benefit by serving as a go-between for the mainstream. As discussed later, women confided that they often found themselves being desperate enough to perform risky sexual requests.

Hustling knowledge of drug availability has increased as an important position in the inner-city drug economy, with drug dealers seeking to avoid long drug sentences for carrying enough weight of drugs to implicate them as distributors. In addition, drug dealers tend to have smaller stashes in more places, and work on a "just in time" business system, in which they try to sell what they have for the day rather than risk stashing it overnight. This makes the women's roles of knowledge hustlers extremely important as they must know on a daily basis what drugs are available among the various dealers. Clearly the concept of going between for the mainstream is created by the middle-class dependence on high-risk women's knowledge in serving as a buffer between middle-class drug users and drug dealers. In addition, drug dealers benefit from these women serving as go-betweens because drug dealers can limit their interaction with middle-class customers who may be undercover police. At the same time, the women must build a preferred customer base among the drug-using middle class and college students, and often do so by playing on these drug users' fear of being arrested or robbed.

Hustling Knowledge of Drugs

Hustling knowledge of drugs is predicated on one's ability to go between customers and drug dealers as rapidly as possible. Ultimately, women who are successful in this role must be swift in connecting drug customers to where they pay for drugs in one setting and pick them up in another. While watching the level of discipline and concentration it took to go between customers and drug dealers, I remember thinking these are the same skills needed in working a living wage factory job. Other skills that appeared to be transferable to mainstream employment included the quality of customer service provided, as well as the skill of being able to quickly judge whether or not newcomers are actual drug users or are associated with law enforcement. Also in terms of "product knowledge," women keep current on drug availability among multiple small-time street corner dealers.

Women who go between as knowledge hustlers tend to work major streets leading into the Rough. I was able to observe this process over time by hanging out with a client named Yolanda, who respectfully cut one of her sessions short and stated in her deep southern accent, "My customers be coming right around this time." I knew she serviced the middle class, but I did not know the details. She explained,

> You know a lot of them be on they job. You be surprised, girl, doctors and lawyers do dope. . . . Don't want to be seen and if I sell them ten dollars and tell them it's thirty dollars. And I make sure I get them something good to keep them coming back. . . . They give me twenty dollars for going to get it.

Over time, Yolanda came to trust me and allowed me to hang out with her on her corner. Watching Yolanda allowed me to learn the inner workings of the idea of "going between for the mainstream." She has been shooting heroin since she was nineteen years old, and at forty-two, she easily looks well over sixty-five. One day I was hanging out with her when she cut our conversation short, explaining that it was time to get ready to watch closely for her regulars, to keep rival knowledge hustlers from moving in on her customer base. Yolanda's method of hustling knowledge began with asking people if they were looking for her nephew or cousin, which was a code to determine which drug dealer they may prefer. A few minutes later Yolanda was on the corner pointing out people and making connections. She collected money, but she never gave them drugs, as actual distribution was the job of someone else, known as a "runner." The role of the runner is discussed later in this chapter. In any case, it is within this setting that I came to see the typical heroin user as a white middle-class individual driving a luxury car and having the appearance of just leaving a professional job. Yolanda hustled knowledge for approximately twenty customers in about ten minutes as I watched from a porch she left me on when she took to the street. After servicing her customers, Yolanda came back to the porch and continued educating me as she pulled out her own drug paraphernalia and proceeded to inject heroin. Once she injected, however, she was less talkative, and the outreach worker who was hanging out with me prompted me that it was time to go. As we drove back to the HIP House, the outreach worker scolded me for staring and said I should act more "normal" when seeing people shoot drugs. What he didn't understand is that for me, I was acting "normal," and in fact, while I had seen people smoke marijuana, it dawned on me that the only time I had ever seen anybody smoke crack, toot powdered cocaine, or inject drugs was on television or in the movies.

Part of hustling knowledge of drugs may include running drug packages from the place where drugs are stashed to resupply the drug dealer on the corner. Package runners must have a level of trust and rapport with drug dealers that is a step up from being a knowledge hustler. This job of running packages had generally been reserved for younger males in the neighborhood. However, now that the juvenile justice system is handing down tougher sentences for first-time youth offenders caught running drugs, school-aged youth are seen as more of a liability because they attract unwanted attention of social service providers. While some youth continue to work primarily in the evenings and on the weekends, drug-using women who gain the trust of drug dealers take on the responsibility of "running packages" during the day. Kawana, who runs packages for her sister, describes how the process of running packages could result in longer periods of work if she smokes crack before paying for it.

> [My sister] came in there and said, run this package down to Big Man for me. And he'll look out for you when you get there. I don't ask her for nothing. I be owing her too much from packages. When she out there working I'll bring customers to her and I come up on stuff like that. Every now and then she might see me looking real stupid and say, here, get these four sacs and bring me back ten dollars or twelve dollars.

Another runner describes how running packages can end up being an all-day job if business is good. According to Sharon, "[Drug dealers] get me running back and forth or say can I give this to such and such. They'll give me something to make me some money. But I just don't be out there on the corner, hollering at people." As Sharon ex-

plains, she sees herself being a step up in the drug-dealing job hierar-
chy as a package runner in comparison to the knowledge hustlers who
interact as go-betweens for the mainstream and the drug dealers.

Other drug-using women in the neighborhood make additional
money or gain access to drugs by "renting drug paraphernalia." For example, Janice keeps an extra straight shooter used for smoking crack
cocaine and rents it out to people who have either lost their drug paraphernalia or who have jobs and choose not to have drug paraphernalia
on their person as they travel to work on the bus or risk someone finding it on the job site. So women like Janice lower their risk for HIV
infection by making money renting out their drug tools. When I asked
her how she makes extra money, she described this process.

> I just be right on the steps. I work alone. When I say work, I mean
> I stand there and wait on a li'l hustle. Wait on somebody who
> want a shooter. Wait on somebody to get off work that need a
> shooter.

Hustling knowledge of drug availability and running packages can
be dangerous, especially when women leave the community with potential customers who promise to share drugs with the women outside
the Rough environment. Other drug users attempt to cheat women out
of promises of money or drugs if they provide knowledge or go get
the package for them. Still, some women have become the victims of
cheap thrills of men. In the case of Dorothy, she hustled her knowledge of marijuana to some college students from a nearby college
community. Dorothy's dilemma is described below:

> Some young guys asked me to show them where some weed
> was . . . but once I had gotten the weed and came back they
> wanted to renege on it which was alright with me. I didn't have
> no problem with that, but for some reason they didn't see it that
> way. And he was like, bitch get out the car. And he told me not to
> look at him. And I had heard that so much when I seen people
> get killed when the person not wanting you to see their face.
> And I was really scared. The knife was really sharp. I can re-
> member that so vividly right now just like it was today. It was so
> sharp and I just knew that those young boys were high and we
> were down in a secluded area. We were in a secluded area and

they were smoking. And I was high. And I was so scared. And I had dope on me. And I had money on me. It was just the fact that those were young kids and I wanted to fit in with that crowd. He pushed me on the car and then snatched me back off the car and told me don't look around. 'Cause he was sitting in the front seat. I could never see his face, but the li'l old red boy and another boy I was sitting in the middle of and so I never did see his face. I never did. Him and the li'l red boy kinda got to arguing and he told him to get back in the car. So he got back in the car in the front and the li'l red boy still told me, he say, don't look back shorty. He say, just start walking. I didn't look back, but I was still scared. 'Cause I was thinking they may shoot me or something. I was still scared. When I thought I had enough room. I took off and I think that's the most scariest I've been.

Women serving as runners put themselves in dangerous positions as knowledge hustlers when they take money from individuals and don't come back with the drugs they promised. Women typically attempt this trick with newcomers and with white drug users in the Rough. Johnsie described a time when she brushed with danger as she tricked a newcomer out of money.

He gave it to me to go buy him some heroin. I came back. When I came back, you so sick you want this stuff so bad now. I didn't spend the money right then 'cause I really wanted to know who he was. When I came back it was three other girls at the car with they pants down and shirts up in the air and he was just sticking money all in them. I'm like, whooo. He giving this money away like that. Then you get, one of the girls gets in the car with him and so I'm checking it and seeing what's happening, so I'm 'a test you, I'm 'a run to the corner and try to stop. You like, I'm stopping you, and you ride right past me and I'm like, this marked money . . . I'm looking. This marked money. That's what I'm thinking. They looking at me like, what wrong with you. I didn't never tell nobody how much I had. Never. But that girl. I sat up there on that corner before I spent any of it. That girl came back and she had 'bout three hundred of them. I'm like, you know that might be the police right there. That might be the police.

Two days later that cracker came back. He came back looking. I say, I wonder do he recognize me. He kept riding and looking at me. I say, damn, I hope he don't pull up in that car and shoot me. I'm scared now. But he left his own money. He left it.

Other women provided stories of times when the drug user did not make good on promises to share drugs in exchange for the knowledge of drug availability. Valerie describes how sometimes hustling knowledge or drug paraphernalia still may not result in getting drugs or money as some individuals use the women's services and try to avoid paying.

I mean like just for instance I take a trick to go get some [drugs]. And he don't wanna take care of me for going to get it, or he probably wanna use my shooter. And don't wanna give me nothing. I ain't had none in about two days. I been dranking.

Valerie shows how drug-using women become even more desperate when their attempts to hustle simply knowledge do not end with them getting drugs or money. As she alludes to, in such a desperate situation, women may end up accepting very risky sex work in order to make up for the losses associated with attempting to hustle knowledge of drugs and having individuals drive off without paying.

Janice, who prefers to hustle knowledge, acknowledges that there is a thin line between hustling knowledge and putting oneself at risk for high-risk sex. As Janice describes below, each episode of knowledge hustling could involve negotiating whether or not a woman is willing to accept offers to gain access to additional drugs or money by going to "party" outside the Rough.

When I say I hustle with dope boys, I mean like I done been around them so much. I may know somebody that come through and they may want ten more sacks, spend hundred dollars or more. And I may have a certain li'l dope boy I go to that I already know gone look out for me when I go. Plus the one I took, the one who money it is, they gone look out for me. Plus the dope boy is gone look out for me. Then I got some hustles where these old low down men in the street be trying to use me. I'll overcharge them for dope. So they be like, you going with me. You gone do all this. I go get the dope and come back. Say they give me fifty dollars. I ain't spent nothing but twenty-five dollars. Twenty-five dollars still in my pocket, plus they gone have to give me some for going to get it. So when I get back to the car, they say, I thought you were going with me. And I'll say, I seen my mom or I seen my boyfriend. I wanna go but, damn. Keep me from going through bull, 'cause I already know, when I say low down, I already know they trying to use this little dope to get me to do anything they want. If I can avoid it, God knows I'll avoid it.

Hustling Knowledge of Sex

Similar to hustling knowledge of drugs, there are women who prefer to hustle their knowledge of the sex trade. Just as individuals from middle-class neighborhoods seek to avoid going deep into the Rough for drugs, men seeking sex who may or may not have a co-occurring addiction to drugs often pay for the knowledge of sex. In this way, women are able to find others who are willing to perform sexual acts they seek to minimize or avoid all together. However, when pushed, several women admitted that (1) if the price is right they may end up servicing the client rather than finding another woman, and (2) if they are desperate on a particular day, they may participate in sexual activities that they would otherwise try to avoid.

"Makeshift madams" are very much a part of hustling one's knowledge of sex. Makeshift madams are women who opportunistically match men with women in the neighborhood willing to perform specific—often higher risk—sexual acts. Sometimes, these women may take the man on as their own customer, but if the woman is on her menstrual or is not feeling mentally or physically healthy, then she will find another woman—preferably one who has provided her an opportunity in the past to date one of her regulars or promises to do so in the future. Women who are full-time sex workers rely on women who interact with male drug users to hook dates. Sharon explains, "Young women will be out there in the street and they might want a friend or something and I might get a friend for them but then they'll pay me for introducing them to somebody."

Peaches is an older drug user who does not work as a sex worker. However, through the makeshift madam process, Peaches has several women she can call on to meet the sexual requests of drug-using men.

> I have never worried about buying [crack cocaine]. I did whatever didn't require me to have to sell myself, or give nobody no blow job. I always knew where to go get a girl that was willing to do whatever somebody wanted her to do and I was gonna reap the benefits.

Perhaps the most risky moneymaking scheme within the sex trade is the concept of "conversating to avoid dating." This phenomenon centers on women's belief that they can talk a man out of drugs or money without actually having to have sexual intercourse or perform oral sex. Women referred to this as having a gift of gab. For example, Peaches stated, "I have the gift of gab. I talk my way through a lot of situations." Dorothy elaborated on using conversation to avoid dating.

> For me, my thing was I had my own little thing, the gift of gab. I could talk. I had a good conversation. I could talk people out of what I wanted. You know manipulation was my thing. It wouldn't so much about the sex, because for me I already knew that sex wasn't what it was about. It wasn't about sex, 'cause every man I had ever been with, they always paid more attention to the dope than they did to me. So, that just let me know it wasn't about me, it was about the dope. When you get through talking he will be done forgot he asked you for the pussy.

Lois's gift for gab is enhanced by her above-average looks, well-manicured hair, impeccable dress, and smell of perfume. She prides herself on being able to set herself apart from other women on the crack scene. In Lois's estimation, men give her drugs because they like being in the company of well-groomed women even if she doesn't have sex with them.

> I run my mouth. I run con games. I tell men, you know you going to get high so you might as well spend your money now. 'Cause you be around females you not going to get what you want. You be around the guys you get what you want. If you dressed nice;

your body clean and you smelling nice and your clothes clean. They going give you what you want and all the time they hitting on you. You just tell them that I'm not like that. Over half of them respect you more and will buy something for you.

Women who are not as physically attractive as Lois are able to use their gift for gab to gain access to drugs or small amounts of money that keeps them from having to have sex with men. Valerie, whose appearance is more typical of mainstream society's image of a crack user explains.

I know a lot of folk. I can stay right up there at that plaza and that liquor store and folks that I know that I ain't seen in a while or whatever, and then folks just, you know, I just know a lot of folks. It ain't about tricking all the time. A conversation will take you a long way. Like folks I done went to school with, or some relative I ain't seen, or some good friends I ain't seen or just some people just tight with me. And then sometime I can go get them some weed or whatever and they throw me something.

Michelle's gift of gab is used after she has collected money for sex work, but before the sex work is performed. Her strategy is to talk to men while they smoke crack. According to Michelle, after he smokes crack, he is no longer interested in sex or he can't get an erection. Because negotiating a time frame for sex work is part of the process, Michelle charges the individual an additional amount of money in order for him to remain in her room once his time is up. She attempts to continue doing this until the man is completely out of money.

Other women are up front with the fact that they do not intend to do sex work, while serving as a companion for men who smoke crack. According to Karen,

A guy say, you wanna kick it? I say, I ain't with all that oral sex. He say, I ain't talking 'bout that. He like for me to talk dirty to him while he hit it. When we got through, he still gave me fifteen more dollars.

In this case, Karen was able to use conversation as a way to get drugs and money from a man who knew up front that she did not want to engage in intercourse.

Hustling condoms as a commodity is key to hustling one's knowledge of sex. For various reasons, many individuals choose not to carry condoms on their person. This increases the value of condoms, particularly when community-based health facilities are closed. As such, at night and on the weekends, condoms can be sold for one or two dollars. In terms of condom sales, women tend to target men whom they believe are hiding from their families the fact that they solicit sex, as such men avoid carrying condoms. Other women target men who do not want to have condoms on their person because they can be used as contraband evidence of intent to prostitute.

Women admitted stocking up on condoms they collect from the HIP House. According to Dee-Dee, "People come get these condoms free. I sell them to them . . . Most of 'em sell 'em." Dee-Dee was the first person to alert me that the "free condoms" from all the various HIV prevention outreach programs were being sold. I was frustrated at first, and even angry that the women would sell something that could save their lives. I was expressing my feelings to an outreach worker who stated that no matter how many times a condom changes hands, it eventually gets used, and thus someone potentially is protected from HIV infection. Moreover, the women who sell condoms use the money to buy drugs and thus bypass high-risk sex. Others confided that even when they have condoms, the process of negotiating with Johns to use condoms can be overwhelming. Also, women were still concerned about condoms breaking or running out of condoms.

Once I learned the condom trade after dark and on the weekends, I began asking women more up front about selling the condoms on the street that they get for free from the project. At first Karen responded emphatically, "No." But she paused and changed her response to "I have." However, she went on to explain the times when she has given them away for free.

> My other sister, she come over there, she spent the weekend and she had used two or three. I keeps them around my house anyway. If somebody give you a dollar for a condom, yeah I'll do it. I ain't had sex in a while, so they just still 'round the house. Then, I have a sixteen-year-old son and he stays in them too. 'Cause if I say, boy, don't you go out there and have no sex, what I look like telling a sixteen-year-old. Like PeeWee, the one that stutter like this, Ms. Karen I ain't ain't got no change. He stutter

when he talk. Here Baby, come and get the condom. Come and get it. I be knowing what he want. Like I say, I don't half sell them, but if they need them and they offer you a dollar, that can buy me a soda.

It was clear that HIV prevention outreach programs are visible and active during normal business hours. However, the sex trade doesn't really heat up until after 6:00 p.m. At this point, condoms are sold; and if people choose more drugs over safe sex, they make decisions not to buy condoms, and thus put their lives in jeopardy. Condoms need to be consistently available for free in the evenings and on the weekends.

RENTING SPACE

Over time, women have learned to avoid "crack houses" as the most dangerous of all settings in which to smoke crack. They described the typical crack house as "filthy and nasty," with fleas and rodents. Women stated that they were so stressed from watching the goings and comings of others in this environment that they did not really enjoy the high. So, they have learned over time to reserve a few dollars for, or share their drugs with, individuals who lease an apartment, in order to have a safe space to smoke and potentially avoid having to turn even more desperate sexual acts to get additional drugs or money to remain in the crack house.

As some women with houses in the Rough need income to pay rent, they charge women a small cash fee to use their houses for drugs or sex. Such women are known as "the house manager." For example, Martha is a house manager and has an apartment in the Rough that serves as a safe haven for working-class individuals who are not afraid to come into the Rough, but who don't want to risk being robbed by young thugs who stick up people in the community for cash. Therefore, they come to Martha's house and give her money to go get drugs from her contacts. According to Martha, she buys the drugs and reaps the benefits, as she tells them the drugs cost substantially more than what the drug dealer charges her. Martha describes her role as a house manager.

In the morning time when people were knocking on my door, I was smoking. People that I get high with. They come to the house and knock on the door and come in and they get high. I am going to get high again with them. When they ain't got nowhere else to go and hit, they'll come and knock on my door. They are friends. The ones that I get high with. Some mornings I let them in, some mornings I don't. If you want to hear the truth, I want to get high too and I didn't have no money to get the dope with; they had the money so I let them in. Sometime it be ladies with they man and they come in and say this the house person. They might give me a sack of crack and maybe five or ten dollars just to be in there. . . . It's some folks come to my house be spending twelve and thirteen hundred dollars. And sometimes I go get them some big dope for less money. I keep the rest of the money in my pocket. So, when they leave, I might have about two or three hundred myself.

Peaches also has an apartment in the Rough, but her clientele is different from Martha's. Peaches provides a place for people from the suburbs who are afraid of being seen in the heart of the Rough purchasing drugs. Just like Martha, however, she overcharges them for drugs and keeps the money.

They come over to my house and I go get it for them. Then I beat them out of all they money. The nickels were so big. I could buy one nickel and make four sacks and they think they dimes. And they be as happy as I don't know what. They be saying, go get me two hundred dollars worth. And on Friday I'll have five or six of them come by there. And every day they'll come.

Just as people rented safe spaces to smoke drugs, there are women who have arrangements with other women to rent rooms to service tricks during the day, while children are at school. Again, similar to the drug scene of middle-class individuals coming to the Rough at lunchtime and right after work, I observed several tags from neighboring middle-class counties—some with baby seats in the cars—coming to the Rough and getting sexual services. For the women who do not smoke crack themselves and have been able to maintain their low-income housing, they make a living by renting rooms in their house to sex workers. Allison explains how she used her friend's house to service her dates. According to Allison, "I got a friend's house over there and I go over there, throw her ten dollars . . . and just gone and use her room."

SHOPLIFTING

Shoplifting among the women was discussed as a key way to get money for drugs. High-risk women who shoplift must have the cooperation of others in the channel supply line, as goods must be quickly converted to cash in order for the women to get money for drugs. Shoplifting designer goods, jewelry, and baby clothes to be sold at reduced prices allows women to serve as buffers for others in the neighborhood. In addition, the women who revealed that they are heavily involved in shoplifting did not participate in sex work for various reasons. On the one hand, they were older women who may not have been as attractive as some of the other women. In addition, several of the women who chose shoplifting over sex work had been raped or had a close encounter with rape. For example, Martha had a bad experience the very first time she took to the streets to solicit sex work. After narrowly escaping from a man who had a knife to her throat up until the time he tried to put the condom on, Martha vowed never to attempt sex work. Instead, Martha relies on shoplifting to augment her disability check. Martha explains how women with addiction problems go back and forth to jail for shoplifting, but rarely get an opportunity to access drug treatment while in jail for this crime.

> I have problems with shoplifting when I get to smoking like that. I'll get ready when the last one gone and I can't think of nowhere else to get no more money, I'll get ready and go on downtown and go in a store and steal something . . . 'cause I just got out of jail the eighth of this month for that same thang.

Johnsie stopped turning dates because she was going to jail too often in sting operations, and escaped two potential rapes in abandoned buildings. Like Martha, she has resorted to shoplifting.

I do a lot of hustling. I boost. I steal out a lot of stores. You go in
the store and steal them people stuff and you take and sell it on
the black market. You got people that run these little stores, they
will buy the merchandise from you and put it into that store as
long the store that you steal from don't have they name on they
product. Like if I go into Kroger. I steal Sensor razors. As long
as it don't have Kroger on it, they will pay me five dollars for
each sensor. And I was good, I was stealing like ten every time
I grab. I might stand there and keep my eye on everybody and
steal 'bout seventy of these things. I come out the end door. Ain't
no buzzer. Walk right out it. Then I go to a fencer. A fencer will
buy all this merchandise. He be waiting on me too. Johnsie, what
you got today? Cartons of cigarettes, perfume, soap, deodorant,
all that. He Indian. They put it in they store and they send it back
home. They say a box of pills, Tylenol, over in they country cost
fifty dollars and it's hard to get medicine. So mainly that's what
they wanted. I could get ten dollars for them Tylenol. I would
just go in there and wipe it off the shelf. A whole thing. Just
wipe it off the shelf. I would just stand there and look and see
where them buzzers was at. Ain't no buzzers on them, I just
swoosh, wipe them off. Zip it up and go to that door and act like
I'm looking at the sales paper and soon as somebody come in
that door I come out. See ya. Walk to the drink machine and buy
a soda and be gone.

As Johnsie asserts, she takes a chance on stealing items from larger
chain stores and sells them to smaller neighborhood convenience
store owners. While Johnsie gives a story of the store owner claiming
to send these products back to his poverty-stricken country, I am inclined to believe that these items are being sold at his store in the
Rough. While I did not ask questions, I did visit several of the local
convenience stores in the Rough and observed a variety of items that
these women are able to shoplift and resell to store owners in the
Rough.
Several women shoplift with their steady partners. The women
help serve as lookouts and cover-ups, and also return items for cash
refunds to stores that allow this policy for "customers" that have no

receipts. Pauline confided that as we were talking, her partner was preparing for a shoplifting spree.

> He hustling. They boost stuff. And he get down. He bring in five
> or six hundred dollars a day. He go get anything. Go in stores.
> And come out with everything, everything. Anything you want
> and bring, he gone bring it. Clothes, shoes, socks, houseware,
> I'm talking about everything. He fixing to go when I get back.
> He go anywhere. He ain't got no picks. He is good. I went with
> him one time. He just do it. He just go with the flow. But when
> I got back with him, we hit large, 'cause I'm very wise too. He
> gets locks, Home Depot stuff, he get everything. Clothes, socks,
> shoes, I got some brand new boxers out there. They silk.

Carmen's steady partner steals jewelry, but she claims she is no longer part of this hustle. "My old man he hustles. He sells slum jewelry . . . I used to be with him while he sell his stuff. But I don't do it no more. But I usually help him go and steal."

Clearly, shoplifting only works as a way to get money for drugs if women can liquidate the merchandise, which requires some level of cooperation from others who are part of the criminal process, but do not face the same punishment for their role in receiving stolen goods. In essence, if there weren't a mainstream market of individuals exploiting these women's addiction in an effort to pay less for high-quality stolen goods, then the women would not risk losing their freedom by shoplifting.

ODD-JOB HUSTLERS

Odd-job hustles are those in which the actual work task itself is legal, morally upstanding, and otherwise a decent job. However, the job is paid under the table and not reported as income, nor is it taxed at the corporate or individual level. The odd jobs described among the women consisted of providing services to businesses and residents in the Rough community. These women are the worker bees for the underground economy that exploits cheap labor in general, regardless of drug use. Individuals who employ these women as a specific type of cheap labor do not have to pay payroll taxes or provide minimum wage, health insurance, or any of the other benefits associated with working aboveground.

Women described being attached to the home remodeling and rehabilitation industry as odd-jobbers, as several of the houses in the Rough are being rehabilitated. The construction contractors hire the women to sleep at the construction site overnight to protect the property from vandalism and theft. This is especially important when appliances are put in or when construction equipment or supplies are left on site. Other women haul trash and keep the site clean while construction crews work on the buildings. Shanese was able to gain shelter in the house where she performed odd jobs. "I work at this house I'm staying. It was a crack house, but a lady came and she rent it out to a bunch of old men, so that's where we've been staying . . . Clean the yard, tearing down the inside of the house."

Some family members use their high-risk family members as cheap labor in family-run businesses. According to Johnsie, "I got a brother who will take me out to his house and he will put me to work. He build furniture for Carson Furniture. He'll have me do li'l work for him." In like manner, Trina's uncle uses her business skills to employ her as a bookkeeper for multiple rental properties he owns throughout the Rough.

Corie cares for an elderly woman in an upscale community and stopped performing sex work when she began working outside the neighborhood overnight.

> I work under the table, so they don't take out taxes on me. I take care of this lady and I been there about a couple of months. I catch a 5:00 bus in the afternoon. I don't get back home. I stay all night. I don't get back home until 7:00 the next morning. And when I get off the bus you know what I'll do? Straight to the corner, start to drinking. You see then, there ain't nothing there but me. There ain't nothing in my life but me. But that's why I know there's not gonna be nothing in my life 'cause I'm not doing anything about it. I go home, bathe, get ready to go back to work. I'm so glad I got a job 'cause I'm not lazy. I'm not home in the house at night. So that's a typical day for me. North Highland. This white lady, real nice lady. She don't know I do, I don't do

them out there. No ma'am! Maybe she done probably smelled the beer on my breath or something but I takes care of her. If you call right now she give you highly good remarks about me. I do my job. I get paid. Now what I do with my money ain't nothing but giving it to them dope boys.

Corie earns money without putting herself at risk for HIV infection. In addition, because her job requires her to spend the night away from the high-risk neighborhood, she is able to avoid some people and activities that had placed her at risk in the past.

Sunnie narrowly escaped jail time on a credit card theft charge. Once she received probation under the first-time offender act, what could have been an eleven-year sentence for credit card theft and carrying drug paraphernalia ended up being a four-year probation sentence. With very few job skills, a sketchy employment history, and her drug addiction, Sunnie's prospects for a legitimate living wage job were limited. However, she was able to market her people skills and gain under-the-table employment as a restroom attendant at one of Atlanta's hottest nightclubs.

Very few blacks come through but I like the tips. I like bringing home a hundred and something a night. That's what I make to pay my rent. And I pay my rent within those four days. Thursday, Friday, Saturday, Sunday. I work at Sunday's at the 201 Courtland. They keep my supplies. I'm supposed to buy half but I don't do that way 'cause I need. I'm sitting there. Some of the customers there are not nice too. But some are. So I'm there taking the ugly ones and the good ones as far as the lines go and I just give him, like, if I make hundred and fifty dollars, I give him twenty-five dollars of it and I take the rest home. But that's just the way I do it. And he depends on me for getting the other women to work. So I try a few women around the neighborhood but they didn't want to do it.

One of the most coveted odd jobs among the older high-risk women who prefer not to have to compete on the streets for sex work clients, is seeking out older men who live alone and need their "house cleaned." I refer to this group as "the dusting daters" because they clean first, and engage in sex work second. Wanda prides herself on having started her own cleaning service targeting older community members. "I clean houses and take care of old people. That's my day." Mona knows the blocks in the community where single elderly men reside, and she goes door to door trying to find older people who need household tasks performed. Others rely on aging or disabled residents who need errands run to the store or trash taken to the curb on trash day.

Once the women complete the tasks of cooking and cleaning, they then seek opportunities to perform sex for money with older men. This strategy intensifies around the first of the month when these men have their social security check or other retirement funds. In fact, at the time of her interview, Allison was grieving the death of two of her older male customers. "I been working cleaning houses. I ain't been selling too much [sex] and most of them old men. Two of them done died on me. Poor thang. I cried worser than I ever did."

Sharon provides a little more of the details. "I have a friend, he like for me to cook, being by himself and all. He offered me to come and stay with him, but I told him he too old trying to get familiar with a young person like me. . . . I clean good. . . . They give me a check or something. . . . They trust me with they house. Everybody in this game don't steal."

Some women attempt to participate in the temporary service as an alternative to high-risk methods of making money. Gloria described how frustrating this process can be for anyone: Whether or not individuals use drugs, they are all viewed as cheap labor who may or may not get picked for work on any given day.

> I work through temporary services. I do catering, I can remodel houses, finishing drywall. Hey, wherever I can find a job or something at that time, so that when I got off I could smoke my head off. Seventy dollars a week. The reason it's finance is because working through a temporary service I'm not guaranteed I'll work. You might work three times out a week. You might only work one day. It all depends on whose working behind the desk and whose gonna send them where. And they have a lot of picks. Certain people they just send out all the time. Then they got people they send out every once and a while. I don't know what be going on with these labor pools, but I go and I be there at 5:30 in the morning and sitting and waiting, and sometimes I go out and

I might even pull a double. Then on top of the double I might work a couple of extra days. Then sometimes I go out and I might only do one day. Then sometimes I go there, and they don't pick me at all. It's a risk. It's a chance I have to take. But until my system is totally clean from drugs I refuse to go in and put in an application because I know that I'm going to fail the drug test. So I set myself up for that.

Mona describes how some chronically homeless drug users attempt to find lower risk hustles for earning money.

We'd get together and pick up cans. Some of us would pick up cans. That wasn't working and maybe before we'd go to work and we didn't have no money. We'd get together and pick up cans and strip copper. You know whatever was pretty much legit. You go and find copper and strip it. Like copper wire . . . We had big money down up under the bridge. They do this all day. I'm talking they might scrap for two days all night long and then get one big pile and they making fifty to sixty dollars. I collect the cans. You know a lot of people collect cans too. Then at night we'd get together and go get some, when it was cold, go get some lumber. Some of us had jobs where they collect wood. Some would find trucks where they would have wood and they get together and collect wood and they chuck some of it down on the side and we'd all take it and haul it up. You know, everybody was pretty much together doing something so we all could survive.

Another odd job for women in the Rough that have houses is that of providing household services for other women. For example, women in the Rough that are living on the streets or are loosely attached to rooming houses rely on house women to wash and iron their clothes, provide a hot meal, take a shower, or even sleep for a few hours for a nominal fee. As Dee-Dee explained, this is one of the most frustrating odd jobs to pursue because the women want these services on credit or would rather pay with drugs.

I say, "Don't ever offer me no drugs. If you got a dollar to give me, you give me a dollar and don't ever think that I'm gone do drugs with you. I'll iron your clothes. I'll wash 'em. You can take a bath, but if you can't do it in cash don't say you got me 'cause it's nothing else you can do for me."

These narratives confirm that women deliberately seek ways to earn money in ways that lower their risk for HIV. However, in the end, the women discussed how they ultimately balance high-risk sex and other hustles. As Allison explains, "juggling multiple hustles" is a more accurate description of the daily reality of making a living in the Rough. "I'm working right now and selling this thang [sex]. Together, that's what I'm doing, and hustling and tricking people." Janice shared a perspective on how hustling knowledge is constantly tempered with performing high-risk sex. "I learned to hustle my knowledge now and not my body. But I'll put my body down if it worth it now."

Women who smoke crack and are detached from the workforce are part of a larger group of individuals exploited for cheap labor. Because most of society believes that good jobs at every level should be reserved for law-abiding citizens, these women continue to lack wide-range networks of advocacy and social programs aimed at helping them become gainfully employed (Gentry, 2004).

The women in this study highlight how their mainstream customer base for designer goods and access drugs serve as strategies to earn money and lower one's own risk. In this way, as we examine the moral lives of the women who steal, we must also be willing to critique the lives and behaviors of mainstream individuals who can afford to pay market price for goods, but who choose to purchase stolen goods from drug-using women. I am by no means stating that drug-using women should not be punished for stealing. However, just as with teen pregnancy, society blames girls for getting pregnant as if this is an act they can commit alone. In like manner, women who steal only do so because they have individuals cooperating to purchase stolen goods.

Drug-using women who hustle knowledge of drugs and sex to the middle class are seen as villains who lure middle-class drug users into getting hooked on drugs (Gans, 1994). The movie *Traffic* highlighted this idea and showed a dramatic change in how crack cocaine impacted our society; prior to *Traffic*, we had a "New Jack City" image of the crack cocaine problem in America as exclusively confined to inner cities and young thugs with no respect for life and community.

Thus, labeling drug-using women as villains who supply middle-class America with illegal substances provides society with a scapegoat for how youth, who otherwise would not be exposed to drugs, gain access to them (Gentry, 2004).

Scapegoating extends to institutions that shift the blame. As a result, some of the responsibility for the existence of crack cocaine in the first place—poverty, slums, unemployment, poor schools—is taken off the shoulders of elected and appointed officials. According to Gans (1994), the availability of institutional scapegoats both personalizes and exonerates social systems. In addition, the blame is removed from a failed economy and shifted onto the individuals' shortcomings. They are exploited by an underground economy that cheats them out of stability and benefits that are afforded mainstream America (Gentry, 2004).

In examining their unique experiences, I came to understand that even on the margins, these are creative women who find a way to build on their strengths in seeking alternative moneymaking strategies and tactics to avoid high-risk sexual behavior. However, there is no evidence-based HIV prevention intervention that focuses on "moneymaking skills building" but rather they all focus on condom use and negotiation skills building. This keeps women safe for a very limited time. However, there is a need for a combined structural and behavioral intervention that focuses on helping high-risk women who choose to exit the sex and drug community altogether.

PRINCIPLES TO GUIDE ECONOMIC-FOCUSED HIV PREVENTION INITIATIVES

Despite their individual circumstances, women shared a common sentiment: They hate turning dates and hate running up credit with drug dealers. Whether they choose to continue using drugs or are seeking a way out, all women expressed a desire to be economically self-sufficient and have a steady income that does not put them at risk for HIV infection. A greater understanding of legitimate ways women can make money can be incorporated into behavioral interventions as an economic empowerment component. This may result in some women cycling out of high-risk moneymaking strategies as they gain knowledge of and access to other means of survival. HIV prevention initiatives tend to focus on helping women stop performing sex work or selling drugs as high-risk moneymaking activities. However, there are very few structural interventions that help women replace the income they may lose, from the sex work industry in particular, by adhering to HIV prevention strategies. These women are limited in many ways in gaining access to living wage jobs, as many have spotty work histories, criminal records, lack of job references, and cannot pass drug tests, which are increasingly required for even minimum wage jobs (Sumartojo, 2000; Holzier, 1995; Fagan, 1993).

Even if most of these women were drug free, almost all would remain part of the cheap labor pool because of other structural and individual constraints (Sumartojo, 2000; Holzier, 1995). Therefore any attempts to stop using drugs as an HIV protective factor can only be successful over the long term if women can find a way to sustain their basic living needs outside the crack economy and more solidly connect to the working-class community (Boyle and Anglin, 1993).

As HIV prevention programs tend to focus on personal empowerment, there is a continued need for appropriate economic empowerment modules for high-risk women. By appropriate, I am referring to the idea that if a key component of risk reduction includes ending one's participation in sex work and/or drug selling, then there must be a practical solution available for how to replace the loss of income. "Appropriate" also implies that women must have at their disposal access to job readiness resources to help them with resumé preparation, interview skills, self-esteem building for rejection management, dressing and grooming for job interviews, providing job leads relative to their education and skills level, and providing a letter of reference for women who complete workshops. Appropriate economic empowerment also means facilitating volunteer or training opportunities for women who have been chronically unemployed to build marketable skills toward gaining access to a living wage job. HIV prevention coordinators can make "keeping the job" or "after you get the job" seminars part of HIV prevention maintenance, including addressing time management, money management, and coping with difficult bosses or core workers as boosters to help women remain on jobs longer as a way to enhance commitment to HIV prevention. Finally, helping affected women clean up their criminal records can be a meaningful module toward getting a better job in the future.

This chapter highlights the ways in which drug-using women build on their strengths and skills to make money in ways that lower their risk for HIV infection. However, these women's dilemmas in being treated as cheap labor due to their drug addiction and chronic detach-ment from the mainstream labor force needs to be understood at a macrolevel. Specifically, we need to examine the political, economic, and social processes that are at the root of these women's economic exploitation. In essence, they are a subgroup of a growing class of indi-viduals labeled "undeserving" in our society, allowing us to normalize their economic exploitation based on their own high-risk behavior. Herbert Gans provided a framework for understanding how these women's drug use, while a personal dysfunction for the women them-selves, is actually a positive function in our existing socioeconomic system. Because so many benefit directly and indirectly from drug-using women's labor and dilemma, our society has less of a motiva-tion to address their problems (Gentry, 2004).

Poor, addicted, drug-using women have been exploited in the crack cocaine economy since the onset of this epidemic in the early 1980s. For example, in the early years, it was common to read news stories detailing the ways in which women had been used as "mules." Women caught trying to smuggle drugs inside their bodies could ex-pect a sentence of between four and six years, but sentences of up to fifteen years were not unusual. While some of these women were the intimate partners of drug dealers, others were women who risked their life and freedom to repay their debts to drug dealers who al-lowed them to run up high drug tabs. Women were known to swallow drugs by the hundreds of grams and then to pass them biologically upon returning to the United States. Some were not lucky enough to make it back, when drugs exploded in their stomachs, killing them in-stantly. Thus, exploiting drug-addicted women for dangerous jobs in the crack cocaine economy is nothing new. However, what has been underexplored in the literature is drug-using women's attempts to make money, but to avoid the consequences of high-risk sex and drug-selling activities as means of gaining access to drugs.

High-risk women's increased risk for HIV must be contextualized as part and parcel of social policies aimed to appease and benefit main-stream middle-class America. Social policies such as Welfare Reform and Urban Renewal, which eliminated large numbers of women from the welfare rolls and from public housing, have forced them into the streets to make money in the drug and sex trade—two of the most lucrative enterprises existing in inner cities across the United States. Paradoxically, if these same women contract HIV, they have a better chance of regaining all the benefits they lost as chronic crack addicts, including housing, disability, medical care, drug treatment, and alterative support groups and social networks.

Chapter 7

Religiosity in the Rough

I used to feel real bad going to churches and eating. I know that there are so many churches and they have so much to offer to homeless people . . . I used to go get clothes and food from the churches. So, I'm grateful to God for Christians.

Dorothy, a 41-year-old recovering crack cocaine user
and former crack prostitute

Dorothy provides a rationale for why HIV prevention researchers and activists must remain committed to partnering with urban-based churches located in the heart of high-risk communities. Today Dorothy is recovering from drug use and is no longer homeless or performing sex work, and her experiences with church reminds us that this social institution has untapped potential as a collaborative partner in meeting the basic needs of high-risk individuals.

This chapter is grounded in the black feminist theme of structure and agency as a way to explore possible roles and activities for churches located in inner-city communities where high-risk women live and engage in high-risk behavior. As part of this study, I spent some time on the weekends observing people and high-risk activities. During my observations, I noticed that the churches in the neighborhood not only attracted individuals for worship services, but also for volunteerism. After the first weekend of observing churches in action, I began to inquire about the women's interactions with the various services churches provide in the community.

In exploring a more effective role for the inner-city church in HIV prevention among high-risk women, I examined the women's narratives of their social networks, everyday lives, and past lives, gleaning

Black Women's Risk for HIV: Rough Living
© 2007 by The Haworth Press, Taylor & Francis Group. All rights reserved.
doi:10.1300/5784_07

information that may indicate some aspects of the role and meaning of church and religiosity in their lives. The social typology that emerged is that of "churched" and "unchurched" women. Churched women can be described as those who grew up in the church and continue to attend. This category also includes women who did not attend church growing up, but have become associated with a church as a tactic for coping in a high-risk environment. The unchurched women are sub-typed as those who attended church growing up, but who no longer attend church as adults. Also, women who didn't attend church growing up nor attend church now are part of this group.

There were four dominant themes among the women identified as being "churched": (1) having positive past memories of their church experiences, (2) currently attending but not fully participating in church, (3) using pastoral counseling as a way to cope, and (4) going to church to gain motivation to maintain the changes made in sexual and/or drug use behavior.

THE CHURCHED

Positive Past Memories of Church Affiliation

Women who grew up in the black church recalled their past memories of their church experiences as youth. For most women, going to a black church in the local community was an extended family ritual. Some of these women participated in the youth choir and had relatives that were preachers, motherboard members, or deacons. Doll recalls the positive reinforcement and public praise she received when she decided on her own at eight years old to join the church in front of relatives and neighborhoods.

> I joined the church in 1987 by myself. Because my grandma was the type of person that's not gonna make you get baptized 'til you get ready. The first Sunday when they asked [if anyone wants to join the church] I got up and I walked down and joined the church by myself. My grandma just burst out and started crying; her, my mama, my daddy. All of us were going to church then. The pastor stood up and said, now baby, what is you come up here to do? I say I came to give my life to God. And you should have seen my grandma.

For some, the church provides social organization and a source of stability in an otherwise chaotic and dysfunctional childhood. Their biological parents did not attend church; however, they found community mothers and a source of morale and familiar role models. Daisy also recalls fond memories of church attendance. "We got to Sunday school. Go to church. We go up to my daddy's Squeeze In. We'd leave Sunday school and go up to the Squeeze In and back and then come home." Dorothy became more involved in the church to help her cope with parenting at an early age. "My mother died when I was fourteen. I had four healthy children. And I didn't know anything about parenting. And that's when the church came into play for me."

Janice grew up in the church, continues to attend church for food and worship service, and sees God as the key to her future. Janice describes how when she was around twelve, some women picked her up from her housing project and took her to what she called a "little bitty small church." "This lady taught us these little songs. Every Sunday me and my sister sang in church. We sang *Another Day Is Gone, Jesus Will Fix It, Trouble In My Way.* That was the good days."

Earlier, Janice had described her upbringing as one with a lot of turmoil, including domestic violence and parental alcohol abuse. As she reminisced about growing up in the church, it was apparent that this weekly worship activity served as one source of stability in an otherwise unstable environment. Janice continues her ties to the church as a high-risk individual. According to Janice, "I go up in churches all the time. I go to churches that have them free breakfasts. I may go and get the 'Word' first. I believe in the Lord." I asked Janice about her future, and her response was rooted in her belief in God. "I'm picking my head up for God. God got something planned for my good." Janice, who grew up in the church, provides a typical narrative for how women with positive past memories of church remember this social institution in their otherwise chaotic lives. As Janice discusses, in the midst of domestic violence, parental alcohol abuse, and poverty, weekly church attendance served as one source of stability in an otherwise unstable environment. She goes on to say that based on that positive experience, even as a chronic crack cocaine user, drug seller, and opportunistic sex worker, she continues to associate with churches as part of her present cool-out strategy. In addition, Janice considers a relationship with God to be part of her future plans. So, clearly a faith-based approach to risk reduction would be appropriate for women like Janice who have positive past memories of church, presently associate with churches, and articulate dependence on God for their future.

Currently Attending, But Not Fully Participating in Church

Women provided several reasons why they feel comfortable attending church as high-risk individuals. In general, church members are kind to visitors and extend a level of social graciousness and heartfelt hugs and comments that can be encouraging to women who experience high incidents of maltreatment by members of mainstream society. In addition, they appreciate not being under pressure to disclose their high-risk behavior. Gloria, whose father was a minister in her hometown of Detroit, joined a church in the high-risk community in an effort to reconnect with her spiritual roots. When I asked Gloria whether or not there was a targeted program at the church for drug users, she explained, "I feel real embarrassed telling you this. I go to church. The baptism and the whole nine yards. I don't know if there is a program or not."

Karen uses church attendance to help her regulate her cool-out time from her drug use to help her body rest, as she is on dialysis. "I smoke [crack] mostly on the weekend. I have my dialysis out the week. I mostly [smoke crack] on Friday and Saturday. I go to church on Sunday."

High-risk women attended church, but very few actually joined churches. While they did not discuss why they stopped short of joining, my hypothesis is that becoming a member takes on another dimension of responsibility and accountability. Once a person joins a church, there is pressure to begin the "sanctification process," which often means adherence to strict biblically-based and not-so-biblically-based rules and regulations governing one's lifestyle and behavior.

Using Pastoral Counseling As a Way to Cope

There were several women like Pamela who attend church and look to the pastor for counseling. Despite this pastor's lack of knowledge of crack cocaine use and subsequent risk for HIV, he attempts to provide Pamela with a message of hope for what she is experiencing. Pamela also is able to approach her pastor without the red tape associated with seeking out traditional counseling. "I sat down and talked to the pastor and he made me feel real positive. He said you going through something right now. He said I can feel it and you don't even have to disclose what it is, but you going to be all right. And that made me feel real good."

Women who did take the next step in moving from attending church to becoming a member discussed using pastoral counseling as an alternative to traditional twelve-step programs. Wanda has substituted traditional AA meetings with pastoral counseling.

> I go to counseling with my pastor. I think that's the best thing to do rather than them AA meetings 'cause I get spiritual healing with my drugs. To me, getting off these drugs is really talking to somebody. My pastor will sit there for five hours and just listen to you talk. He say just get it out. I'm gonna continue to go to my pastor. To me that's my AA meeting.

One of the benefits of pastoral counseling is that there generally is not a waiting list to speak with pastors at smaller churches; however, most are not trained in addiction counseling. Dorothy highlights how her pastor provides pastoral counseling. "My pastor told me, he say, put your hand on your head. He said, now take it off. He say, that's where your problem is, in your head."

Some inner-city churches have developed spiritual-based drug recovery programs; however, it was unclear from the women's narratives the extent to which drug abuse counselors integrate HIV prevention messages into their recovery plans. What is noticeable is the women's feelings of empowerment as they discussed their connection with these various drug recovery ministries. According to Mona, "When I was in the Ministry they showed me that I was a queen and I did not have to settle for second best; did not have to be mistreated by nobody else if I did not want to. Thank God for the Ministry."

Using Church Worship As Motivation to Maintain Risk Reduction Strategies

For high-risk women who have completed some type of risk reduction program, the church serves as a place for sustaining and maintaining risk reduction goals, particularly when women are discharged from an HIV prevention program. Several women expressed that hearing messages of encouragement empowered them to continue making positive changes. Closely related to the idea of motivation is the use of church as a place to build and rebuild one's self-esteem. Rebuilding self-esteem is an important task for women involved in drug abuse and facing stigma and discrimination on multiple levels.

Motivation to maintain is represented in Lisa's narrative about how church attendance gives her motivation to maintain the behavioral changes she committed to as part of the HIV risk reduction program. Lisa tells how she uses the church as an institution of motivation.

> Like your mind get on the wrong path and you go walk in somebody church. It helps me think about certain things. But, as far as physically help me with my problem, no. But it helped me think. It helps me to push on and say, keep doing the right thing. Keep paying the rent. Keep paying the bills. Keep taking care of your children.

Similarly, Lois maintains her motivation by going to church and praying.

> I been going to church and praying. I'm proud of myself. I just pray and keep on going to work and go home and play with my grandbaby and I listen to the tape I got from church and I tell myself I can do it. The only thing I got to do is pray and leave the dope alone.

Wanda's narrative provides a glimpse of the strengths and challenges associated with the church as a collaborative partner in HIV prevention.

> I want to get fully, fully save. The biggest thing I want right now is I want God to be the head of my life. I want to be save. If I get

save like I suppose to be, then none of this will be a problem. This time last year, it was rough. But now I can sleep at night and don't have to worry about where am I going to sleep; what am I going to eat. Am I going to have money tomorrow, am I going to have some clothes tomorrow. Do I have somewhere to wash? I'm trying to get my life together. Just getting off drugs ain't everything. 'Cause I can get right back on drugs.

Specific strengths are that women are able to have sources of support and interaction at times when HIV prevention case managers may be unavailable, as well as the church's ability to provide a safe environment within which to maintain one's commitment to risk reduction. At the same time, churches' general lack of knowledge and capacity to provide traditional case management for high-risk members may limit their ability to effectively reach and retain individuals who make some initial positive behavior change.

Churches are proving capable of addressing issues women are most concerned about that may serve as barriers and facilitators to HIV risk reduction programs; for example, simply washing clothes for homeless women and providing food. As Mona asserts, first meeting women's physical and practical needs enhances the church's ability to meet their spiritual and mental health needs. Mona describes how a church focused on the physical and spiritual needs of the homeless.

I didn't get to go to the church to Lithia Springs where the white people keep coming to. I didn't get to go Sunday, but I went up to the day shelter. Ever since, this would have been my third Sunday. But I still got a little church. But God bless me I'll make it Sunday. They white people, but God don't have no color. They give me spiritual food and physical food.

THE UNCHURCHED

There were four dominant themes among the unchurched women: (1) church as a negative past memory, (2) depression, (3) closely related to social isolation, and (4) not ready to change one's high-risk behavior.

Church As a Negative Past Memory

The narratives of unchurched women who have negative past memories of church suggest that there is a need for both faith-based and community-based interventions with no references to church, as some women have made up their minds that church cannot be part of their lives. When I asked Portia about her church attendance, she exclaimed, "My mother's a minister. I ain't going to church so she can talk about me. No, no, hell no!" As a churched youth myself who attended church on Sunday for two services, Wednesday prayer meeting, Friday night joy night, and Saturday choir rehearsal, I can identify with her. Portia's mother, a minister, nagged her to go to church when she was growing up and today scrutinizes her every behavior as being sinful and against her Christian upbringing.

Two women described a negative memory of church affiliation as a child. Punkin recounted how she was molested by a deacon who took her to church and offered her money to perform household chores.

> I been to church before, but I never been in one since I got molested by a deacon. The church over there by Thomasville we used to go to. Well the deacon they stayed next door to us. He used to have me come over there and wash his dishes and stuff. That's when he used to do it; he still paid me though. I didn't tell nobody except my brother. My step momma wasn't gone believe me no way until he did the same thing to her. That's when I stopped going to church period.

Punkin believed the reason no one intervened and she didn't feel empowered to report this deacon's crime is because she was already sexually active. According to Punkin, "I had already been laying with any and everything since I was ten." Lolita's bad memory with a church leader who is also her grandfather was described earlier in the chapter on family relations.

Depression

Martha, who doesn't attend church, described being depressed and using more drugs to cope with depression, and being more depressed because she uses drugs and is caught in a vicious cycle of drug use and depression. According to Martha, "I believe if I had a counselor where when you get depressed instead of drugs, you call them. 'Cause I have trouble with depression. Any little thing bothers me. Then I'm gonna either go get me a can of beer or take me a hit."

Pauline discussed her current state of depression. "Well right now I'm having a hard time trying to regain the process of being able to be strong again. Trying to get my kids back and, um, right now I'm living a miserable life, very miserable."

Closely Related to Social Isolation

Corie represents a large portion of women who are unchurched today but actually grew up in the church. She talks about having values and morals, but continuing to engage in high-risk behavior. She says she prays but even that doesn't solve the social isolation problem, which leads to loneliness and to getting high as a way to cope with the feelings of social isolation and loneliness.

> I have values and morals, but I rather go up there and beg up on somebody than to just do anything for it. I don't feel it no more. It's not exciting anymore. 'Cause I pray even though I get high and drink. And I'm lost. I'm lonely and I get high.

In addition, unchurched women were more likely to describe themselves as loners or lonely. For example, according to Sunnie, "I'm my own person. I be by myself. I don't group with them. The only time I group with women is like this or down there at the [HIV Intervention Center] where we used to have our meetings. That's it." Frankie echoed the feelings of loneliness that emerged among unchurched women. "I don't even have people that I socialize with. I don't even have visitors."

Not Ready to Change One's High-Risk Behavior

In general, women classified as unchurched were less motivated to change their high-risk behavior. In fact, the study included ten women who made no attempt to change their high-risk behavior and all of them were also classified as unchurched. Tomeka is one of several unchurched women who explained that she is not ready to change her high-risk behavior. These women had a range of reasons for not associating with churches, from having been sexually molested by male church leaders to simply not believing that organized religion will benefit them. According to Dee-Dee, "I do everything I can to stay out of church. Because ain't nothing in them churches but hypocrites." Mattie gave further insight on why some women may avoid churches. "When I see you [preachers] doing what everybody else doing and you're preaching, you're not practicing what you preach. Like if I see a preacher out picking up girls on the street, what can he do. Like this one that got this rooming house at the top of hill he was busted down there." Sharon, on the other hand, did not have any particular reason for not attending church, but simply stated, "I don't go to church on Sunday. For me, it would fall apart if you kept trying to force me to go." Still, other women like Allison view the church as part of a bigger strategy to change one's life.

> If I was going to a treatment house I couldn't come back this way. You can't come back to the same environment. You got to go where people are going to work every day. People that's going to church. People that care for you. You got to go somewhere and get with some people that's bettering themselves, and get your morals and self back together.

A THEORETICAL FRAMEWORK FOR UNDERSTANDING POTENTIAL ROLES FOR INNER-CITY CHURCHES IN HIV PREVENTION

The findings in this study suggest that faith-based organizations in inner cities may be untapped resources in delivering HIV prevention. In general, the women in this study have confirmed their willingness to interact with inner-city churches, but these institutions lack evidence-based HIV prevention programs.

Based on the women's accounts of their own experiences with churches, I developed a theory of the relationship between church affiliation and response to church-based HIV prevention intervention, which is summarized in Table 7.1. The first premise is that women who attended church growing up and attend/interact with churches

TABLE 7.1. High-risk women's current ties to faith-based institutions.

N = 45		Currently interacting with a church in the community	
		Yes	*No*
Attended church growing up	*Yes*	Most likely to respond to faith-based centered HIV prevention intervention (*n* = 10)	Uncertain of their response to faith-based centered HIV prevention intervention (*n* = 12)
	No	Highly likely to respond to faith-based centered HIV prevention intervention (*n* = 7)	Least likely to respond to faith-based centered HIV prevention intervention (*n* = 16)

today are most likely to see faith-based strategies as an important part of their HIV prevention. The second premise is that women who did not attend church growing up but attend now are highly likely to believe faith-based strategies will work for them in some form or fashion. The third premise is that we need more research on women who attended church growing up but no longer attend, with respect to their willingness to participate in a faith-based HIV prevention program. Finally, women who have no past or present ties to churches are least likely to respond to or to benefit from faith-based HIV prevention programs, suggesting that there remains much work for community-based programs not affiliated with churches.

PRINCIPLES TO GUIDE FAITH-BASED HIV PREVENTION INITIATIVES

In assessing the potential impact of inner-city churches on HIV/ AIDS prevention and intervention, there are several strengths that are underdeveloped. Not only do churches have a biblical basis to be compassionate in their service to the poor and homeless, but they also have long-standing community presence and can serve as effective outreach and retention partners in HIV prevention. Church members and leaders typically build trust and rapport in a way that complements HIV prevention program needs to recruit and retain high-risk individuals in multiple-session interventions. Also, churches have capacity to serve at various levels, which can be transformed into program sustainability as HIV prevention program funding periods end. These strengths, however, exist within the context of long-standing challenges associated with the churches' conservative doctrine (Gilbert, 2003).

Just as the case with other churches, inner-city churches follow a doctrine of serving the less fortunate with compassion. Within the inner-city communities, the application of this Christian principle alone has resulted in high levels of trust and rapport among community high-risk dwellers, many of whom may have been associated with these local churches during their childhood and adolescent years and continue to depend on their support in getting their basic needs met— hence community outreach as a strength. Also, churches have space that often goes underused during the week when HIV prevention programs would potentially want to operate in the community.

One of the main barriers to fully integrating inner-city churches as collaborating partners in HIV prevention hinges on the general lack of understanding of core elements of harm reduction and risk reduction models among church ministry leaders. To be fair, churches have been at a disadvantage in not having access to faith-based and evidence-based HIV prevention programs disseminated in turnkey boxes that are often used by community-based organizations.

The FAITH-model for faith-based HIV prevention capacity building is intended to be low cost and less intimidating than traditional evidence-based models (Exhibit 7.1). HIV prevention program coordinators can use the FAITH-model as a tool to help bridge the gap between churches and HIV prevention by suggesting some useful activities and Bible references that add validity to the suggestions. While there is no scientific evidence to support the effectiveness of faith-based guidelines for a suggested HIV prevention format for churches that want to help high-risk women, I have developed this model based on my own training as a minister-in-training at the Women's Institute of Ministry. It fuses my knowledge and practice as a behavioral scientist with my understanding of key biblical principles that support core elements in the transtheoretical change model. At a minimum, the FAITH-model can be used to legitimize a role for faith-based organizations in HIV prevention and serve as a way to increase the possibilities of churches' inclusion in community collaborations (Jackson and Reddick, 1999).

EXHIBIT 7.1. The FAITH-Model for Faith-Based HIV Prevention Capacity Building

Fellowship
- Churches can sponsor fellowship activities with HIV prevention programs targeting high-risk African-American women.
- Biblical Reference: 1 John 1:3—That which we have seen and heard declare we unto you, that ye also may have fellowship with us and truly our fellowship is with the Father, and with his Son Jesus Christ (*The Holy Bible,* King James Version, 1979).

Awareness
- Church members involved in Health and Wellness, Outreach, Women's, Youth, and Christian Counseling Ministries should be educated on AIDS and HIV prevention strategies.
- Biblical Reference: Hosea 4:6—My people are destroyed for lack of knowledge: because thou has rejected knowledge, I will also reject thee (*The Holy Bible,* King James Version, 1979).

Issues
- Churches that have women in the ministry can sponsor spiritual modules that focus on helping high-risk women identify with women in the Bible who suffered from various mental and physical health problems.
- Biblical Reference: Luke 8:43-48—And a woman having an issue of blood twelve year . . . and he said unto her, Daughter, be of good comfort: thy faith hath made thee whole; go in peace (*The Holy Bible,* King James Version, 1979).

Transformation
- Churches can complement HIV prevention programs using public health behavior change models that promote behavioral modification in stages, starting with a change of mind about one's risk factors and protectors.
- Biblical Reference: Romans 12:2—Be not conformed to this world: but be ye transformed by the renewing of your mind, that ye may prove what is that good, and acceptable, and perfect, will of God (*The Holy Bible,* King James Version, 1979).

Hope
- Churches can serve as an additional resource for women entering the maintenance stage of their risk reduction goals, which is particularly important for women residing in environments where they run the risk of reengaging in high-risk behavior with other members of their drug-using social networks.
- Biblical Reference: Romans 12:12—Rejoice in the hope, be patient in tribulation, and continue to pray (*The Holy Bible,* King James Version, 1979).

While many universities involved in HIV prevention research conduct their studies among high-risk individuals in high-risk communities, these researchers often close out their project without sharing their findings and without developing a sustainability plan, which could include churches, to maintain parts of the program that the community grew to depend on. Much of the current literature that references church involvement in HIV prevention focuses primarily on continued barriers of the black church as an institution in general and as a collaborating partner for specific HIV prevention programs. In this way, both scientific articles and anecdotal comments emphasize a discourse of what the church will not do as part of HIV prevention. HIV prevention researchers should conduct an "interest assessment" among churches located in high-risk neighborhoods. Such an interest assessment should distinguish between various target populations, as it is clear that the church in general services the needs of the poor, women, and children in ways that complement adherence to traditional HIV prevention strategies.

Moreover, an interest assessment differs from a needs assessment in that an interest assessment is developed to explore the church's interest in meeting various HIV prevention needs among high-risk women. In the past, HIV prevention program coordinators have approached churches with their own needs, which are generally centered on condom distribution during church activities. As the women in this study confirm, their HIV prevention needs encompass more than just the need for condoms. However, HIV prevention researchers should be sure that having the church meet HIV prevention needs among high-risk women does not compromise the church's doctrine.

Another way in which HIV prevention researchers and program coordinators can help the church is by providing pastors, Christian counselors, Health and Wellness Ministry, Women's Ministry, and Outreach Ministry participants with basic HIV prevention strategies. These strategies can be incorporated into existing church models for reaching and engaging high-risk individuals that are either already part of the membership or among those encountered on the streets during church outreach activities.

Also, churches have capacity to provide space that could be used for individual, group-level, and community-level interventions. In like manner, families who attend inner-city churches and have one or more high-risk family members can benefit from the church hosting a support group to help these families cope with the behaviors of their family members. Activities may include educating the churched family members on how to deliver HIV prevention messages to their high-risk family members.

Because social commentary is a key type of sermon, HIV prevention researchers can provide ministers with HIV prevention facts and research findings pertinent to the black church and the black community to use in their sermons. Such guidelines might include suggesting that the facts and figures be used in sermons in recognition of World AIDS Day or Black HIV Awareness Day.

There remains a need to help members of churches involved in community outreach ministries to understand the key components of behavioral change theory (Bandura, 1994). The following information can be used as part of existing presentations to churches aimed at increasing their involvement in HIV prevention programs. Table 7.2 helps HIV prevention program coordinators demonstrate how public health theoretical models are compatible with—not contradictory to—biblical doctrine.

TABLE 7.2. Stages of change and biblical compatibility.

Stages	Stage definition	Relevant biblical verses
Stage 1 Precontemplation	Earliest stage of change, when some individuals are unaware of the full extent of consequences associated with their high-risk behavior.	*Jeremiah 18:12* And they said, There is no hope: but we will walk after our own devices, and we will every one do the imagination of his evil heart (*The Holy Bible,* King James Version, 1979).
Stage 2 Contemplation	When individuals begin to think about the risk associated with their behavior as well as evaluate for themselves the potential rewards and losses associated with changing their behavior.	*Philippians 1:6* Being confident of this very thing, that he which hath begun a good work in you will perform it until the day of Jesus Christ (*The Holy Bible,* King James Version, 1979).

TABLE 7.2 *(continued)*

Stages	Stage definition	Relevant biblical verses
Stage 3 Ready for action	When individuals who intend to change their high-risk behavior begin to set definite goals and priorities that will help them change their behavior.	*Deuteronomy 30:19* I call heaven and earth to record this day against you, that I have set before you life and death, blessing and cursing: therefore choose life, that both thou and thy seed may live (*The Holy Bible,* King James Version, 1979).
Stage 4 Action	When individuals take direct steps to change their behavior and are able to do so for at least thirty days and up to six months without reverting to old high-risk behavior.	*Philippians 4:13* I can do all things through Christ which strengtheneth me (*The Holy Bible,* King James Version, 1979).
Stage 5 Maintenance	When individuals have been able to successfully change high-risk behavior for a period of six months or more.	*Galatians 6:9* And let us not be weary in well doing: for in due season we shall reap, if we faint not (*The Holy Bible,* King James Version, 1979).
Stage 6 Relapse	When individuals revert to old unhealthy behavior.	*Romans 7:19* For the good that I would I do not: but the evil which I would not, that I do (*The Holy Bible,* King James Version, 1979).

Chapter 8

Reducing Risk in the Rough

First of all, [the interventionist] she helped me to eat more. I regained and maintained my strength by eating, stopped staying up, and try to use more protection, try to get off the streets, and she tried to help me get in rehab. I was almost there.

Pauline, a 32-year-old crack cocaine user
and sex worker

The women for this ethnographic study were selected from among 400 women who participated in a larger intervention, which used quantitative methods to analyze women's risk reduction outcomes. For several reasons, however, the accounts of women's changed behavior gleaned from their narratives may differ from the larger quantitative study's finding. First, I used language often reserved for qualitative research, such as "tell me about life after the intervention," or "tell me about your experiences with drugs and condom use after the intervention." Such different methods of inquiring about changed behavior led to different responses (Patton, 1990). Also, many of the women who were motivated to change during the first two years of the HIP intervention may have relocated to other neighborhoods. While I attempted to include some of these women, it would have been difficult to locate those known to have left the Rough in the early years. Therefore, the women I found in the Rough to participate in the ethnographic interviews may disproportionately represent those who had a harder time changing risk behavior because they remained in the high-risk neighborhood or returned after a short time away. In addition to discussing the intended change behavior traditionally associated with risk reduction, I have attempted to contextualize the

doi:10.1300/5784_08

"other" changes made by these women on the margins, which they count as risk reduction. There are four discourses that emerged in discussing how women reduced their risk for HIV infection in the Rough: (1) leaving the Rough for drug treatment, (2) practicing safer sex, (3) making other positive changes, and (4) making no changes.

LEAVING THE ROUGH FOR DRUG TREATMENT

Women who left the Rough for drug treatment or rehabilitation programs were perceived to be the most successful and serious in terms of lowering their risk for HIV infection. However, many returned to the Rough after participating in programs ranging anywhere from three days of detoxing to six months of longer term treatment.

Janice attempted drug rehabilitation; however, she checked herself out after three days in a detoxification program, when she was about to be placed into a longer term program. I asked her why she left, and she stated with all sincerity, "The devil." She described how she gathered her personal belongings and rushed out to catch a bus back to the Rough. Her skin was burning and she felt extremely nervous over the three days she detoxed. In her opinion, "That ain't no rehab!" I asked her what would be the perfect rehabilitation program. Her perception of the perfect rehabilitation program consisted of a "home-like" environment where she would go about daily life "just not smoking dope."

Janice's idea of a drug rehabilitation program that resembles home is a common theme among the women in this study. They resent the stigmatizing public treatment facilities because in their opinion too many people are there to avoid prison sentences and are not seriously committed to making behavioral changes. Several women commented they could find just as many drugs in treatment as on the street. Janice represents a viewpoint among drug-using women that the current structure and processes associated with public drug treatment do not fit their needs. It is much easier for men to be successful in the "dormitory model" of housing for drug treatment, where someone cooks and cleans for them, and which does not accommodate small children. Women, however, prefer a greater sense of privacy, would rather cook their own meals, and care for their children while they recover. They also like the social intimacy found in small women-only groups as a way to discuss issues that pertain to them without being overshadowed by men.

Women who were homeless or raped in the Rough were more motivated to enter drug treatment as a way to gain access to housing and get counseling for the trauma associated with being homeless or raped. Ka-Ka, an attractive 36-year-old recovering drug user, experienced both homelessness and being raped in the Rough. She admits she came to the Rough because she believed she could make money in this neighborhood as a sex worker. Ka-Ka remembers getting raped after ignoring the advice of a woman who lived in the Rough.

> This lady told me "don't go in any isolated areas." It was night-time and I just wasn't thinking. I took him up through a shortcut and it was real dark, vacant houses. I mainly stayed around this area. [I was approached by a trick who] didn't look right. I said, "come on, let's go." Then he just grabbed me and pulled me in the house. He got me in the chokehold and I couldn't get up. And I guess he'd seen that he was killing me and he came up off me. He was definitely killin' me. Basically after that, I just went to my friend's house, took a bath, was cryin', telling him what happened. He wanted to have sex. I told him, "I ain't havin' no sex with you. I wind up stayin'." When I woke up, my body was just aching all over. I had bruises and everything. I walked up to the [HIP House]. And that was the end of that. I stayed 'til [the outreach worker] got here.

Ka-Ka moved to a suburb of Atlanta with her steady partner after getting kicked out of two drug rehabilitation programs. Currently, she is working two jobs and attends aftercare meetings. In addition, she now has a five-month-old grandchild and is reengaging with her family.

Mona, on the other hand, returned to the Rough after six months in a residential-based drug-treatment program. After things did not work out with her steady partner, she eventually began turning dates and smoking crack again. Like Ka-Ka, Mona recalls the night she slept on the HIP House doorstep, waiting until a member of the staff arrived and drove her to a detox center. This resulted in Mona going into what she calls "the Ministry."

> The intervention project has really helped me get myself together and go into the Ministry. One day I had went out and been drunk all night. I made it right here on the porch. When [the project director] got here I was drunk sleep. I say, please help me, please help me. I don't know what to do. Will you let me take a shower? She go on give me something to eat and freshen me up and I went to sleep and was alright. After that I went into the program, the Ministry.

Mona left "the Ministry" after a few months to share an apartment with her steady partner, but soon began drinking and drugging again. Mona has a clinically diagnosed mental health illness that may need more professional and medical attention than can be provided at a faith-based drug rehabilitation program. While the faith-based program has many strengths in terms of encouragement and helping women gain a sense of hope for their situation, women with mental disorders need additional services.

Dorothy is one of the few women who took advantage of an opportunity to gain access to drug treatment through the court system. In fact, most women were adamant that they were not willing to participate in jail-based drug rehabilitation programs because it was forced on them. They didn't feel mentally free to really focus. Dorothy was arrested in a crack house. She asked the judge to send her back to jail rather than release her to return to the Rough. This plea for help resulted in Dorothy being placed in a treatment program under the Drug Court program, which offers drug-using, nonviolent offenders an alternative to jail for breaking laws such as shoplifting, trespassing, and possession of small amounts of drugs. As Dorothy attributes her ability to maintain long-term change to moving out of the environment, she confided that she did not even feel comfortable coming back to the Rough to be interviewed because of the impact of "triggers." Thus, after the interview, I personally drove her out of the Rough even though she insisted she had a bus pass and could get back on her own. While I was curious to see her new home, I was more concerned that Dorothy get out of the Rough as quickly as possible and not have to pass her "old playgrounds."

Getting women into drug rehabilitation programs as HIV prevention proved effective in helping women in the Rough set short-term goals toward positive changes in their lives and high-risk lifestyle.

HIV prevention programs should include a discussion distinguishing long-term and short-term goals to help women understand the consequences associated with returning to the high-risk environments. Some women sincerely believe they are strong enough to live in the Rough and remain drug free, as this is the only environment some have ever known. Others return because they have no other place to go upon being released from drug treatment programs. Still, others return to show their former acquaintances how well they are doing since leaving the streets. Regardless, HIV prevention programs targeting chronic drug users should include a module on the pros and cons of reducing risk in Rough-like settings. This may provide women with a greater incentive to seek alternative living arrangements after leaving inpatient drug rehabilitation programs.

Many of the women in this study were court ordered into drug rehabilitation to protect their unborn fetus or after giving birth. For example, Valerie admitted that the first times she went was to avoid jail and get her children back after giving birth to babies who tested positive for crack in their systems. Now that she has had an opportunity to talk to people whom she believes are truly committed to helping her, she would like to try drug rehabilitation without being forced into a program. In the meantime, she has begun to attend a weekly HIV prevention program run by another community-based organization in the neighborhood, and likes the fact that she can talk about her problems and "let herself go" without anyone judging or forcing her to make changes based on what she reveals. In fact, I still have Valerie's social security card and birth certificate that her now-deceased mother gave me to hold should she decide to go to drug treatment.

Like Valerie, Johnsie wants to go back to drug treatment, having been put out in 1997 for breaking what she referred to as an unnecessary rule, consisting of not speaking to the men in the program. She expressed that if drug-treatment programs took on a home-like approach comparable to the HIP House, more women would be inclined to commit to such a program.

Martha set up an appointment to go into drug rehabilitation, but the morning an outreach worker came to drive her to the facility, Martha would not answer the door. According to Martha, "They referred me to go to rehab and I been hardheaded and I won't go. They made me an appointment to go into the rehab and I changed my mind. I saw her pass my door and I closed the door and window." Even though she did not go into drug treatment, she recalls her short-lived clean time.

> I'm going to be honest and tell you the truth about it. I started coming here in October, and I started doing a lot better 'cause I stopped smoking [crack] for two months. I started doing a lot better. And when Christmas came around I messed around and started back. I never went out seeking it; my friends they will come to the house and put it in my hand, you know, and to an addict it kind of rough to turn it down 'less'n you truly got yo' mind made up saying, this is it. I guess they thought they were doing me a favor. I believe they thought they were giving me something for Christmas.

Based on Martha's initial enthusiasm and willingness to stop using crack, I am convinced that she may have remained drug free for a longer period of time had she been able to leave the Rough. As it stands, Martha was not strong enough financially and physically to say goodbye to her social network. Even though she made changes in her life, people from the neighborhood still frequented her house seeking a safe place to smoke their drugs. They were accustomed to paying Martha with crack for her services as a "house woman." Thus, having limited income from disability, Martha caved under the pressure of continued visits from paying members of her social network.

Some women in the Rough discussed being in families where others either sell or use drugs, and are also labeled high risk. Women in this group face barriers in that others in their house often remind them of their old behavior by continuing to indulge in it themselves. Often these women are mocked and monitored for signs of low or noncommitment to their goals to behavioral changes. Group intervention has proven effective among social networks that are at risk. This same approach should be applied with families where crack cocaine is used by two or more blood relatives living in the same household.

Since HIV is being widely transmitted in crack houses via prostitution, one direct route to prevention would be to decrease the number of people addicted to crack cocaine. In fact, as it relates to HIV, today's crack houses have become yesterday's bathhouses frequented mainly by gay men undercover from their families, and the family-housed women's dilemma has worsened. Just as with the gay community, these women need a safe place out of the environment to make changes. Unfortunately, public drug-treatment facilities historically were designed to treat heroin addiction and have not been able to adequately adapt their services and approach to rehabilitation to meet the changing faces of drug abuse brought on by the crack epidemic. This has meant that even some women who do make the steps toward drug treatment often are at the mercy of drug programs which are unable to meet their gender- and cultural-specific needs.

While I remain in contact with several of the women in the study, Kawana is the one woman I spent the most time with to date. While I had served as the behaviour interventionist with three women over the two years who were lesbians, Kawana was the only one I located for the qualitative interview. The other two went to treatment and moved out of the Rough. At the end of her interview I asked Kawana where she wanted to be in a year, and she replied:

> In my own place. So, next June so my li'l boy can come and spend the night. I made that promise to him. My aunt say don't tell him things that you are not going to do. I know I'm going to have to disappear again from him for a while, 'cause I got to get away. I got to get away. I would rather go off in some program instead of wasting my time withering away and getting more and more depressed. Having some glasses and a decent job. It ain't got to be decent, just a job that I can get up and go to every morning. I been looking forward to doing this interview for some reason. I guess I wanted to get my side out. I really did. I was thinking about it. Every time I would come in at night since you brought it up to me I would be like, "man this would be perfect." The way I feel right now, this would be good stuff for that interview. Because I want her to really know how it sucks out here you know. So, I'm glad you chose me so I can tell the truth about how I feel about being out there.

After hearing Kawana express herself, I felt moved to commit myself to helping her achieve her one-year goals. At the end of the interview I asked Kawana what she needed from me. She replied, "I need you to just keep in contact with me from time to time. So, it's not like after this you just leave me right?" To that I responded, "No, what do you want me to do?" She then asked me to help her get into treatment. I had no idea where to begin, but I asserted that I would try. I was concerned that she may have been seeking treatment to avoid a possible jail sentence for violating probation; therefore I insisted that she go see her probation officer first, and then call me after that meeting.

Kawana called as she promised that Monday, and by Wednesday she was in a detox program. I took her there and visited her during the week she was in detox. I braided her hair while she was in the detox program, and became acquainted with two other women (MiMi and Shay) who were her roommates. MiMi was excited because she learned she had been placed in a long-term drug rehabilitation program with an excellent reputation for helping women remain clean for longer periods. I met MiMi's parents that Sunday afternoon, and thought they would be thrilled their daughter was placed in such a great program. However, her father was vocally frustrated because of the fact the detox facility had air conditioning. He didn't care that it was eighty degrees in Atlanta; he simply believed these women should be "punished" and not "treated this good." He became even more agitated as they described how good the food had been over the week they were detoxing. For me, it confirmed the continued confusion and animosity between drug users and their non–drug-using families. Also, I realized the lack of understanding the African-American family still has concerning what exactly drug treatment is, as well as the "criminalization versus medicalization" of women in recovery.

That same day, Kawana and Shay, the other roommate, learned they would be placed in a program with a reputation for being unorganized and disproportionately housed with residents who were court ordered to rehabilitation. Many were still using drugs and selling them in this facility, as some accepted drug treatment only to avoid jail time. Kawana did not want to go and complained about not being placed in the program with the better reputation for women. She shared her detox program discharge papers with me, as she could not read them because she had no glasses. The counselor had written that Kawana would relapse because of the lack of "hindsight." She jokingly remarked that the cause would be lack of eyesight. I purchased her a pair of glasses, and later drove her to the program that would allow her to remain for eighteen months to two years. I went by her grandmother's house to pick up her personal belongings and carried them to her.

Kawana checked herself out of the program after six months and began living with a female partner she met in rehabilitation. Her rationale for moving is complicated; however, she cited several reasons for leaving. First, she was working and had to give her check to a counselor, who gave her some small portion back after accounting for expenses related to living in the drug rehabilitation center. Next, she did not understand why the recovering community warned them against relationships of any kind. Also, she was demotivated by the fact that subcontracting counselors and group facilitators were often no-shows. Kawana was also hurt by the further marginalization she received because she was "not feminine." In her mind, she entered this program to break her isolation, but found herself even more alienated from the other women in the program.

In addition to the pressures she encountered inside the center, she wanted to impress her family and convince them of her capability of being a mother to her son. She also resented the stigmas attached to the institution of drug rehabilitation, and developed a complex of not wanting people at work to know where she lived. However, she expressed the major problem for her was facing the ridicule from men and women who shunned her for revealing that she was a lesbian. She felt betrayed as she initially bought into the idea that this was a safe place to talk. In telling her "I" story in group sessions, she reflected on how her first drug binge in 1989 was to mask the pain brought on by her breakup with her girlfriend who was attending Spelman College, while she attended Georgia State. She believed that after being so honest, some people distanced themselves from her. In her opinion, she could have dealt with the distance, if they had not been so openly mean.

I tried to talk Kawana out of leaving by trying to make sense of the rules that seemed arbitrary as well as her perception of the overall ineffectiveness of the program. In addition, I used my own example of having grown up attending schools in Atlanta, which had the reputation of breeding criminals and teen mothers. I told her how much I did not want to go, but I was stuck in these stigmatized schools. I explained that I could have dropped out, but that would have amounted to making a bad situation worse. My analogy of trying to be successful in poorly run institutions was convincing initially, and Kawana remained for three more months. However, I was no match for the love she had for another woman in recovery, and they planned to leave and set up a household together.

I did help Kawana get a job at Georgia State University in food service, and I helped her find a Narcotics Anonymous lesbian meeting group. She stopped by my office regularly every week to talk and loved meeting any students who were around. She said the university brought back fond memories because she had completed a year and a half of college prior to doing drugs. Toward the end of the semester, Kawana called me and asked if I could buy her and her steady partner a monthly bus pass so that they could purchase Christmas gifts. She promised to pay me back with her first check following the holiday season. About a week after that, she called me to inform me that she and her partner had relapsed Christmas Eve, 2000.

I did not panic, but was extremely frustrated because she had been doing so well. She asked me if was I mad at her, and I was, but I didn't say so because I really wanted to keep my word of being there for her. We talked every day for about three weeks, and Kawana and her partner both decided to go into separate new programs in January 2001. A year later, she asked me to come to attend a meeting where she celebrated one year of sobriety. As of May 2007, when I did the final edits on this book, Kawana remains clean, gainfully employed, and permanently housed in a two-bedroom apartment. In addition, she continues to provide emotional and financial support for her teen.

While Kawana's story is by all accounts a great ending, perhaps Allison more accurately articulates the dilemma facing most of the women in the Rough who have not attempted drug treatment as a risk reduction strategy.

> If I was going to a treatment house I couldn't come back this way. You just can't come back in the same environment. You got to go where people are going to work every day, people that's going to church, people that care for and don't have no nonsense in their house.

Unfortunately for Allison and her cohorts, there aren't enough safe and affordable environments available to absorb women who need a new environment to return to after lowering their personal risk in drug rehabilitation. So for many, they return to the Rough and some are able to remain clean, but for so many others, over time they reengage in the subcultural norms associated with living in the Rough.

PRACTICING SAFER SEX

Dorothy admits that when she first came to the HIP House she did not set goals, but because of the persistence of one particular outreach worker she kept coming back. She recalls how this worker would "hound you to death" and just wouldn't give up on her. Dorothy started using condoms immediately after her intervention began. She explained that after intervention, she would be walking with a sex work customer and would tell him "wait 'til I get these condoms." She had to get aggressive in keeping the customer, however, because many would threaten to find someone else. She would exclaim, "No, you goin' to wait 'til I get these condoms, that's what you can do!"

She was afraid of losing the customer, but was determined to try to practice safe sex. In addition, Dorothy recollected a series of events and circumstances that convinced her that even as a homeless person who was desperate for money, she needed to use condoms. First, she had caught a sexually transmitted disease, and remembered thinking that it could have been worse, in that it could have been AIDS. Next, she recalled that several members of her drug-using inner circle were diagnosed with HIV/AIDS, and she was afraid because she knew she had sex and smoked crack with those same people. Finally, she perceived her weight loss to be a symptom of having HIV infection. These three factors resulted in her having a change of mind by the end of her intervention. Despite initially not wanting to come to sessions, by Dorothy's last appointment she told the interventionist, "I am going to do something for myself. I am tired."

I asked about her present sexual behavior. She explained that she no longer socializes with people who are using drugs, and because of that disassociation, she no longer sees herself as promiscuous. "I just got one sex partner now. That in itself for me is a miracle." She elaborated on the "miracle" aspect of her behavior change by asserting that she believes for her to have gone from using crack at all costs to now being able to look in the mirror is a miracle. "For all the mercy and grace God had for me I'm a miracle." Dorothy attributes going from being absolutely homeless to having shelter and one steady partner to God; she defines it as a miracle. However, there were several steps that she had to take personally in order to change her life. Later, she discussed this process. First, she described how, when she learned that the conversations with her interventionist were confidential, she used this as an opportunity to be honest with herself about the lifestyle she was living. Second, she immediately tried to practice safe sex. Third, she changed the way she thinks about herself and her behavior. Finally, she changed her environment. Thus, what Dorothy refers to as a "miracle" was actually her willingness to take control of her own life and make some changes.

Janice insists that she continues to use condoms since her intervention. She recalls moving from not caring if she had condoms to being more responsible in carrying condoms.

> I learned to stack up on them [condoms]. If I ain't got none in my pocket I stopped him [the outreach worker] and say, "you got some condoms with you?" I hate to walk around without some rubbers. I use them a lot. That changed a lot. I used to didn't give a damn.

Janice also learned to walk away from men who continue to insist on having sex without a condom. Even though she now carries condoms, she still faces the fact that some men simply refuse to use them. I asked her what she does in those instances. According to Janice, "They might say, 'well you wanna forget it.'" She responds to them, "Well yeah forget it then man."

Mona insists that she has increased condom use during sex work, but acknowledged that she does not use protection with her steady partner. She explained that for women who really want to change behavior in terms of condom use, it is easy, because in her perception there are plenty of condoms in the community. I asked her why she felt she was unable to use protection with her steady partner, and she exclaimed that she no longer has sex with him because she caught him in an apartment naked with another woman. She is now on the waiting list to get back in "a faith-based drug recovery program," but in the meantime she takes to the streets to avoid physical confrontations with her partner.

The thought of being further ostracized from the family convinced Valerie to make some changes in her life. She was one of the few women who described herself as having a strong sex drive. The other women downplayed the pleasure they derived from sex from both paying and steady partners, particularly when doing crack cocaine. Valerie, believing she was more at risk from intimate partners, began masturbating rather than having casual sex. "I got to have it. But I use the '3-Supreme' to keep me from getting anything." For Valerie, increased masturbation resulted in lowered risk for HIV, as she avoided unprotected sex.

Tracie did not give up drugs or prostitution, yet she was able to translate her new knowledge about HIV infection into positive action. Tracie highlights that the intervention helped her to change her mindset from being a woman who "prays" that her dates don't have AIDS to making sure she has condoms. When I asked Tracie about her goals for changing her behavior, she explains:

> I wanted to change my whole behavior not just my sexual behavior. Because I know my behavior stems from my drug use. Once I change that then the sexual part is automatically gonna change . . . because in actuality I'm just a one man's woman.

Daisy, who considered herself to be from what she called the "old school," discussed how people from her generation didn't use condoms. Therefore, coming to the HIP House to learn the benefits of condom use helped her. She now uses condoms more consistently, as she has become more assertive in insisting that her paying partners use them. She was one of the few women who found the use of condoms to be so important that she would not sell the condoms to her partners; she provided them for free. She admits, "At first it was hard 'cause I never used 'em (condoms). I never thought about using 'em. I think about it all the time now. I pulled it out and said wait a minute, let me get this first. Put this on and they were alright with it."

Daisy, who has some college education and has worked living wage paying jobs most of her adult life, was disappointed that she did not achieve all of the ten goals she set during her intervention. She recalls, "I think about those ten goals that I had written down that I supposed to be doing. I done some of 'em and some of 'em I haven't done. I got to get back on track." I asked her which goals in particular she felt strongly about, and the two that were important to her included getting a job and going back to school. In her mind, if she could achieve these two goals, then she believes her drug problem would minimize itself over time.

Kawana, a self-reported lesbian who only had sex with men to support her crack use, explains how she approached paying customers after her intervention. "I didn't tell them I was going to practice safe sex, I just did it. 'Cause trying to educate them on the situation—it's just a lot of men are very ignorant to the facts about the education of sex." Kawana recalls becoming more motivated to work toward changing her behavior after learning that she was HIV negative. Like others, she had taken AIDS tests in the past, but never followed up to get the results and posttest counseling. Even at the HIP House, at first she did not want to know her results because she remembered all the chances she took in having unsafe sex. However, once she learned she was HIV negative, she recalls getting focused on changing her behavior in order to maintain her negative status.

MAKING OTHER CHANGES

In addition to the changes women made in their sexual and drug-using behavior that resulted in lowered HIV risk, thirty-six women reported "other" positive changes that impacted their risk for HIV. There were three dimensions of other changes discussed. First, women discussed structural changes in that they improved their housing arrangements and gained access to legal, living wage employment. Second, women changed their interpersonal relationships and exited abusive relationships, at the same time increasing interaction with community-based programs, churches, and their families of origin and procreation. Some entered new relationships that they viewed as more positive and supportive of their changed behavior. Finally, women discussed changes in their physical and mental health, including gaining weight and eating more regularly, as well as increased self-esteem and decreased depression.

Valerie cited several changes in her life since the intervention that may not have been adequately documented in a study designed to measure changes in drug use and sexual risk behavior. "I done changed a hell of a lot since I been coming down here. I don't jump on nobody no more. I don't hang down there [on the corner] like I used to. Basically I be at home." She was happy to take the HIV test, but admitted that she thought she could have been infected. According to Valerie, she remembers thinking, "What would I tell my Momma. What would I tell my daughter? They already treat me fucked up as it is."

Pauline did not report reduced risk in her sexual or drug behavior. However, she vividly remembers making some other changes.

> First of all, [the interventionist] she helped me to eat more. I regained and maintained my strength by eating, stopped staying up, and try to use more protection, try to get off the streets, and she tried to help me get in rehab. I was almost there.

Pauline describes the things that were important to her. Eating and sleeping properly were placed ahead of using protection in her daily life. In addition, Pauline echoed the sentiments of many women in the study in that, just when they began to trust the interventionist and move toward making some permanent changes, their intervention ended. This is not a criticism of the HIP House in particular, but of prevention programs in general. Pauline had two very complicated issues in her life that impacted her willingness and ability to make the measured changes of decreased drug use and increased condom use in the beginning: Her father, with whom she had lived all of her life, died; afterward, her son, whom her father was raising, was placed into foster care. According to Pauline, he repeatedly ran away from foster care trying to get back to his family in the Rough. She feels she fell short of her goals because she was worried about the death of her father and the repercussions it had on her son. After talking about these issues in her first few sessions, she was ready to focus on risk reduction. However, Pauline only had one more formal interview, but did come by periodically to see if someone was available to just talk.

Karen was only able to make limited changes in her behavior, and attributes her "modified" behavior to the intervention. While she did not stop smoking crack, she perceives herself a success in the program because she slowed down. According to Karen, "I ain't gone say I really just stopped. I slowed down through my counseling making me feel good about myself." Karen could not pinpoint changed sexual and drug behavior, but she termed her changes as "the little bitty" ones that are very important to her.

> It's a lot of changes. It's little bitty ones but it's very important to me. My situation with food in my house is real thin. It kinda made me feel bad; much money as I get a month I'm supposed have something in that house. It [the intervention] changed me from not keeping no food in the house to being able to keep some in the house. When I left here and my check had came that day, I made my money order out for my rent and instead of me going straight on to the crack house, I stood right there at the store and bought me some cigarettes and a lighter and I bought some toilet tissue and some house spray and some lunch meat and a loaf of bread, some mayonnaise, bought me a big pack of cookies and I bought me some scratch-offs, then when I got home I didn't have much money as I usually have 'cause I spent bout thirty dollars, forty dollars in the store.

Karen recalls a major consequence of her intense drug use was not having food in her refrigerator. She gets a disability check because of her kidney failure. It is important to note that Karen was enrolled in the negotiation session, which centers on helping the women negotiate with sex partners. Karen, however, is on dialysis and does not "desire to have sex right now." Thus, it appears that the interventionist improvised and focused on issues that were relevant to Karen in a way that helped her develop strategies and tactics for improving her quality of life. Once she began spending more on food and other household necessities, she had less money to spend on crack. Karen admitted that she never stopped smoking crack altogether, but after redefining her personal goals she spent less money on drugs.

While Corie did not stop smoking crack, she stopped performing sex work and began less risky work outside the neighborhood after her intervention. She explains how employment indirectly impacted her behavior.

> I work under the table so they don't take out taxes on me. I take care of this lady and I been there about a couple of months. I catch a five o'clock bus in the afternoon. I don't get back home. I stay

all night. And before I got this job if I needed some money or somethin' somebody come through I put a rubber on and sold some pussy.

Corie is now able to earn money without putting herself at risk for HIV infection. In addition, because her job requires her to spend the night away from the high-risk neighborhood, she is able to avoid some people and activities that had placed her at risk in the past. Thus, she went from "catching whoever comes through" to "catching a bus" out of the Rough.

Lolita reported that she has been abstinent since her intervention because she had pneumonia. Lolita, who has been clinically diag-nosed with mental illness, expressed that she just felt better about herself. According to Lolita, she came to the intervention in the first place as a way of gaining access to someone to talk to about the recent death of her son. She says she had been so depressed and it made her smoke even more crack in trying to cope with the pain associated with his death.

I had just lost my son and I was so depressed. And you know everybody that you talk to don't understand your feeling. You get to say it but they want you to hear what they got to say. So I just need that bullshit out of my damn mind. When I came in here I felt so relieved. 'Cause it was so much pressure off of my mind . . . 'Cause it so loving. I loved it. I could say anything I wanted to say. And I felt very good about myself. When I got back at that house everybody be sayin' that I done changed.

Lolita used the intervention as an opportunity to release the men-tal pressures associated with her son's death. She did not feel she was at risk for HIV/AIDS because she has not been sexually active in what she called a "long time." I probed further because one of the requirements to be part of the study is that women must have smoked crack and had sex within thirty days prior to their intervention. Lolita, who admitted to suffering from mental health disorders, could not recall the last time she had intercourse. Nevertheless, her narrative in-dicates that she benefited from the opportunity to have someone to talk to about her pain. Another family-housed woman, Sunnie, provides an account of how the intervention led to slowing down her crack use.

> At that time I was a heavy user . . . Okay, I smoke crack . . . Okay, I was heavy user smoking . . . I was smoking over two hundred dollars a day . . . Now, I'm down to maybe one sack a day . . . I let that be that . . . They put a great impact there. And they were always concerned. And that meant a lot for somebody to say, hey you guys ought to think about stopping, you know what I'm saying—try anyway. And I done got fat now. When I first started I was skinny. I was skinny. I was wearing a seven to eight, now I'm in a fourteen. So I'm doing good.

Sunnie believed her intervention was successful because she now smokes less crack than before. In her mind, an immediate benefit of slowing down was gaining weight. Many women who smoke crack are conscious about their weight loss because society attributes rapid drops in size with either being strung out on drugs or HIV positive.

MAKING NO CHANGES IN BEHAVIOR

There were nine women who asserted that they made no changes in their lives as a result of the intervention. I wanted to compare and contrast the narratives of the women who did not make changes in their behavior or lifestyle after their HIP House experience. Such an analysis provides HIV prevention researchers with a clearer under-standing of unmet needs among high-risk women. In fact, overcoming the barriers these women face should serve as the catalyst for planning and implementing new HIV prevention programs.

Teresa learned she was HIV positive at the HIP House. For me, the most difficult part of this project was informing women they were HIV positive. I recall there being two types of responses. There were those women whose lack of emotion seemed to indicate they already knew they were infected prior to coming to the HIP House. Then there were the women who I felt were hearing their status for the first time generally, who either cried hysterically or became angry. Once we calmed them down, however, most were receptive to hearing about ways to get help. Teresa's reaction was to become enraged with anger. Unlike others, she refused all help from the HIP House to gain access to HIV care and treatment programs. Thus, it is no surprise that her attitude remained negative about the outcome of this program.

To be fair, many women discussed that they were doing well for periods ranging from one month to a year after the HIP House, but then they returned to using drugs and engaging in high-risk sexual behavior. The women expressed a desire to have a continued counseling program in the community where they could come and talk about anything on their minds, mainly as a way of getting the courage to do what they believe they should be doing for themselves. It is unclear, however, if Teresa would have attended such a support group given her state of outrage. As angry as Teresa was, she was able to articulate a phenomenon that results in middle class black women who are not in the Rough to be at risk for HIV.

> People come through and people up women and payin' us and they get on back with their wife. Nine times out of ten they have condoms. That's all I come through those married men. I don't know why they won't get it from their wife. They'll rather come out here and pay all that money.

In the past, mainstream women who became infected overwhelmingly believed themselves infected from bisexual partners. However, according to Teresa, the trend is now "mainstream" heterosexual men frequenting Rough-like neighborhoods, primarily for oral and anal sex. Many end up having vaginal sex as well. As many men continue to choose women who look relatively decent, Teresa is often chosen over her street corner counterparts because she maintains her appearance. Thus, women like Teresa, who refuse care and treatment programs, continue to service clients who move in and out of "Rough-like" neighborhoods secretly servicing their sexual addiction. In this way, she is potentially exposing large numbers of women to HIV infection who think themselves unlinked to Rough-like activity.

Portia asserted that she only came to the HIP House when the outreach worker explained she would get paid for her time. She laughingly remembered talking to him because she thought he was a potential sex work customer. I asked her about her intervention and she recalls, "I talked about drugs, what I did in my life, my family, then he paid me and I got the hell on." She paused and added, "I came back and I even got my certificate." Getting the certificate means that she completed all her sessions. Many women were proud of the certificate, as it signified to them that they were capable of completing a program. Some women used the certificate to show family members they were connected to a program centered on helping them change their lives.

The one positive change Portia did make was to separate from an abusive partner. While one might argue she had no choice after being evicted from the condemned apartments, the fact that she has internalized the separation as a choice she made is a starting point. In addition, the HIP House intervention did result in Portia getting tested more regularly for HIV, as she had heard rumors that Juicy Fruit had been infected. Portia's sexually transmitted disease turned out to be a treatable one. She attributes her knowledge of getting tested and going back for the results and counseling to her sessions at the HIP House.

Portia, who reported no changes, admits she didn't change because she didn't want to change. She never set goals and only separated from an abusive partner after his family refused to allow her to live with them when their apartment was condemned. She remains in the Rough selling drugs and performing sex work, and insists that changing her behavior is not worth it because it will not result in her reuniting with her children and family.

Yolanda recalls her initial excitement about the HIP House after seeing one of the outreach workers in the Rough whom she knew was in recovery. She thought that if this outreach worker could become clean, then so could she. She recalls trying to get clean over and over again, but it did not work for her. Like Valerie, when Yolanda came to the HIP House she was pregnant. As noted earlier, several women feel pressured to go into a drug-treatment program for the good of the unborn child. Yolanda gave her baby up for adoption and began street hustling again. I asked what part of the intervention worked for her, and she explained that having an HIV test, counseling, and results within walking distance was the best thing about the program because she would not go downtown to the health department. Yolanda is convinced that she has been doing drugs for so long she simply cannot change at this point. In fact, Yolanda actually believed that getting HIV may help her get her life together.

You know I'm out here living this life, they say it come from sharing needles this, that, the other but who knows? Don't nobody know for real but God. So I just asked God to look over my shoulder and hopefully, you know, like I said, if I had it, Lord all I can do is I will get off of dope. That would make me get off of dope and take care of myself.

Yolanda rationalizes that getting HIV may result in her taking better care of herself. Several women raised this point as the public discourse has shift from people "dying from AIDS" to "living with HIV." These women contextualized the impact of HIV/AIDS in their lives as poor African-American women who smoke crack. It occurred to me that HIV infection is one of the few ways that poor drug-using women can gain almost immediate access to drug treatment, health care, housing, disability, food stamps, professional counseling, support groups, and job placement. This is particularly the case if these uninsured women are willing to enroll in HIV drug trial programs, where they may be part of the "treatment" group. So, a poor woman who has been living in the streets for a long period of time may not associate HIV with death, but rather as an opportunity to live a "better" life for at least twenty years in some instances.

Thus, as Yolanda described it, "It's just a vicious cycle!" For poor African-American women who smoke crack, this cycle consists of not having the resources to avoid risky behavior, as social services are denied them. However, should they become infected with HIV, they gain access to the very social services they were denied as poor African-American women who smoke crack. The cycle is vicious in that the women may have been able to avoid HIV infection had they been given the resources earlier.

Chapter 9

Black Feminist Theory As Behavior Change Theory and Practice

Ain't no control. Whatever y'all do ain't nothing gone change. It's gone take a hell of a lot to get a person off drugs. They got to come with some kind of cure, some kind of medicine. But just talking and trying do this and that for them, that ain't lasting.

> Teresa, a 37-year-old HIV-positive crack cocaine user
> and seller, sex worker, and mother of five

Throughout this book, I discussed principles to guide the next generation of HIV prevention initiatives as gender and culturally appropriate high-risk women. These principles are guided by the reality that conditions that lead to black women's risk for HIV are different from other high-risk groups. Moreover, the barriers and facilitators that impact one's ability and willingness to (1) acknowledge and (2) change high-risk behavior are different for black women along a continuum of high-risk factors and circumstances. Despite these differences, HIV prevention strategies continue to support traditional risk reduction techniques that have proved effective in lowering risks among other high-risk groups (Fisher and Fisher, 2000). As the women suggest, their lives are more complex as they grapple with intersecting oppressions and limited choices that are part and parcel of their risk for HIV. In this final chapter, I present a case for using the core principles of black feminism as key elements of an applied HIV prevention program targeting high-risk women.

Black Women's Risk for HIV: Rough Living
© 2007 by The Haworth Press, Taylor & Francis Group. All rights reserved.
doi:10.1300/5784_09

I began this behavior research with the idea that a deeper understanding of the women's everyday lives and decision-making process
would help me understand the core elements of the next generation.
of HIV prevention programs aimed at high-risk African-American
women. At the end of this undertaking, I realize that in order to
change lives you must change minds; and in order to change minds,
you must change hearts; and in order to change hearts, you must understand history. In this way, I am inclined to agree with Teresa, who
in the opening quote is very pessimistic about the future of HIV prevention programs' current capacity to help black women change over
longer periods of time. As she articulates in her own voice, long-term
change must take on a new commitment to engage high-risk women
on a deeper level. For high-risk black women, I am adamant that any
attempt to plan and implement HIV prevention programs not
grounded in black feminist perspective will be limited in its approach
and scope. At the same time, I challenge black feminists to become
more involved in public health research and practice. This is the only
way black feminist theory will be viewed as a legitimate framework
for change in public health. It is our responsibility to provide a methodology for how black feminist themes can shape public health programs in general, and HIV prevention programs in particular. In this
chapter, I apply black feminist themes as the core elements of an HIV
prevention program based on the ethnographic findings from this
study. A black feminist perspective allows these women to speak
about their everyday experiences in order to discover aspects of
changing risky behavior that currently are not included as part of traditional risk reduction programs.

Poor African-American women who use drugs see HIV as part of a
larger problem impacting them and the Rough as a disintegrating community. Collins (1990) has conceptualized these "bigger issues" as a
matrix of domination, referring to the overall organization within which
intersecting oppressions originate, develop, and are controlled. She
further deconstructs the matrix of domination into four parts. First,
structurally, there are laws that allow injustice to permeate our entire
society. For these women, the most relevant are our laws concerning
welfare, drugs, and housing in America. Second, the implementation
of the laws and policies ensure the transformation of racism and sexism from one generation to another. Next, the hegemonic nature of the

social organizations in our society justifies the continued unequal practices of bureaucracies, which leaves marginalized groups depoliticized. Finally, as the women in this study have confirmed, the matrix of domination has a component that absorbs these women interpersonally, as they experience on a daily basis the unequal practices of our major social institutions, including the U.S. legal system, labor markets, schools, the housing industry, and social services. Given the list of "other" killers in impoverished urban areas, keeping a roof over one's head is often a more pressing priority than the threat of HIV. Moreover, the women in this study suggest that the motivation for their changed behavior is less influenced by individual reasons and is more related to concerns for family or significant others.

A key implication for HIV prevention intervention programs is the role of referrals in linking these marginalized women to outside the Rough. The women who made longer commitments to change had help in leaving the Rough via connections to social services that assist at-risk citizens. Those who returned to the Rough were highly likely to revert to the old unsafe practices, while those who remained in residential drug treatment programs or community-based drug ministries, and relocated to more socially integrated communities, were able to continue safe behavior practices. Moreover, gaining access to safe and affordable housing begins to address some of the larger structural issues that place these women at risk in the first place (Woods, 1998).

By incorporating key components of black feminist theory into existing HIV preventions, planners can take a closer look at what works in the lives of poor African-American women who smoke crack when designing more effective programs. One of the key contributions that black feminist scholars have made in sociology is to challenge dualistic thinking. In the case of behavioral change, traditional measures have been "either/or" conclusions. For example, conventional scientific standards for measuring program success limit researchers to conclude that either a woman changed her risk behavior or she did not. Perhaps, black feminists' most radical premise has been their rejection not only of what is concluded about black women, "but the credibility and the intentions of those possessing the power to define" (Collins, 1991a). According to Collins (1991a), when black women define themselves, they clearly reject the taken-for-granted assumption that those in positions granting them the authority to describe and analyze reality are entitled to do so.

Black feminist perspective argues that the "other changes" defined as important by the women should be moved from the margins to the center of prevention intervention for the simple reason that the women themselves focused on them as self-defined successful outcomes (hooks, 1984). Because the women declared these changes as central to their lives, I argue that they should be the basis for building programs that are effective in the lives of at-risk women (Scott, Gilliam, and Braxton, 2005; Ward, 1993; King, 1988).

Traditional risk reduction methods are more effective in the lives of people who have race, class, and gender privilege in our society (Auerback and Coates, 2000). For these women, a greater emphasis was placed on basic survival needs, such as eating on a regular basis, getting steady employment, and securing safe, affordable housing. Once the women saw improvement in their daily lives, they made even greater commitments to increase condom use and decrease drug use. Moreover, the women who made permanent changes were those who were able to change environments—even if temporary—as opposed to changing within the environment (Geronimus, 2000).

Black feminists have consistently maintained that African-American women have agency, and they often use this argument to empower African-American women to act up for a change under current oppressive conditions (Guy-Sheftall, 1995). hooks (1981) argues that mainstream feminism has never emerged from the women who are most victimized by the various oppressions and are powerless to change their condition in life. Thus, black feminism provides a platform for empowerment that includes the voices and perspectives of crack users who are at risk for HIV in high-risk environments.

A greater appreciation for the past and present plight of African-American women will help prevention specialists develop better individualized plans. For example, interventionists need to consider that homeless women who have been deprived of socioeconomic resources may react differently to receiving HIV-positive results than would middle-class persons who have a higher stake in society. Both groups of women may be initially shocked, hurt, angry, or scared of the meaning of an HIV-positive status. Because of the evolving meaning of HIV due to medical breakthroughs, a homeless woman may internalize the meaning of HIV as a way of gaining access to social services she was previously denied. In addition, the meaning of HIV has shifted from a discourse of "dying from AIDS" to "living with HIV," as one can realistically live for an estimated ten to twenty years with HIV, depending on other medical and socioeconomic factors. However, the meaning of HIV among the middle class and the truly disadvantaged over time will differ greatly: One may view it as a loss of privileges, whereas the other can point to some gains in housing, drug treatment, mental health counseling, job search assistance, and access to health care.

HIV prevention intervention planners also need to understand that the meaning of crack cocaine in the lives of high-risk women is totally different than what outsiders might expect (Sterk and Elifson, 1993). For example, in addition to just wanting to get high, poor crack users may view crack as a stress or pain reliever, as many have limited and stigmatized professional counseling, preventive medicine, and health insurance. Thus, risk reduction strategies that attempt to convince crack users of the harmful effects of the drug may not be as successful in practice because of the positive meanings and benefits the crack user perceives she derives from the drug. Therefore, interventions that include sessions about the potential harm of crack cocaine must take into consideration the meaning this drug has taken on among users at various stages in their drug-using career.

In terms of behavioral change via risk reduction, poor African-American women interpret and select for themselves the "slices" of change they will attempt generally based on their daily reality. These "slices" are highly dependent on women's perception of changes they can make within their current environment. Once these women attempt risk reduction, in whatever form, they are likely to suspend actions that are not working, and to rethink and retry those goals they really want to achieve. Moreover, over time they are likely to transform their thinking about risk and risk reduction in light of each interaction in which they are placed at risk and primarily direct their actions based on their unique interpretative process. In this case, the process is influenced by their self-perceived reality of being poor African-American women who smoke crack.

HIV prevention specialists need to understand how poor crack-using African-American women can be both victims and villains in a high-risk environment. Hence, depending on the situation at any given time, they may be "tricked" or they may "trick" others with whom they inter-act. For example, women who trade sex for crack or money may begin their day with condoms, some money, and drugs left over from the previous day. If they have these resources, they are in control of the interactions that take place with potential customers.

If women are not desperate at the beginning of the day, or when-ever they decide to take to the street, they may even be inclined to turn down sex work that appears risky. This includes someone wanting anal sex, wanting to take them out of the neighborhood, or not want-ing to use a condom. They express verbal and nonverbal signs that they are not desperate at this time, and those they encounter will respond to their demonstrations of control. They are also keen at gleaning clues from the conduct, appearance, and attitude of potential customers, some of whom they may know from previous encounters are attempt-ing to get sex without paying. Thus, if they are presenting themselves as sex workers and deliberately hiding the fact that they smoke crack, they may be able to maintain control of the situation.

However, if it is a customer who has known them in the past, he may become frustrated with their appearance of control, as he knows they smoke crack and often perform risky acts for money and drugs. The potential sex customer's patience wears thin when he is not able to get them to act in his favor if he knows that the women are mem-bers of the stigmatized crack-smoking sex workers. This may prompt him to walk away from the negotiation in search of a woman who is willing to meet his price and perform his preferred sex act. Thus, some-times even if these women are not desperate for money or crack, they may change their presentation of "safe self" to maintain clientele.

Some of these women attempt to deceive newcomers to the drug and sex trade out of money and drugs. They do this by taking the new-comer's money and promising to go deeper into the high-risk environ-ment and bring them back the best drugs. Newcomers and non-African Americans come to the edge of the high-risk environment, but remain at the mercy of those who act as go-betweens for the drug dealers. If the women believe the people will not remember them or attempt to find them later, they may never return to give the newcomers their drugs or money.

However, as the day goes on, some crack-using women find them-selves having smoked their drugs, spent their money, and now in need of more resources to get through the night. Thus, they shift from a position of self-control to one of vulnerability. Once others in the environment—potential Johns and drug dealers in particular—assess them to be desperate and weakened, they may approach them to perform again the very risky acts the women confidently declined earlier. It could be the same people making the request or another group of men whose own meager resources only allows them to approach those who are willing to sell sex cheaper than women who may not be using drugs. Thus, crack-using women who present themselves as practicing safe sex may do so during certain times of day. However, a more careful analysis of their full range of activities during the day, week, and month may reveal a self that takes risks at certain times and under certain conditions.

In addition, because of the stigma attached to crack cocaine, even among drug users, many crack users seek to differentiate themselves from the "generalized other" crack smokers. Most crack-using women attempt to avoid such labels applied to crack users in general (crackhead) and crack-using women in particular (crack whore). Some, however, become immune to what others think of them over time and may not react in a way that leads to changes in risky behavior. In essence, they display a presentation of self that makes it harder to implement risk reduction because they put on defensive fronts about their risky behavior. HIV/AIDS interventionists must understand how various social interactions in the everyday lives of crack users may impact behavioral change. These social interactions generally are based on unequal social positions between crack-using women and more powerful drug dealers and sex solicitors in particular.

Drug-using women pass through distinct stages of socialization that draw them deeper into the socially stigmatized crack subculture and may result in more encounters in the high-risk environment that heighten their risk for HIV. For example, a woman who smokes crack is not at a high risk for HIV simply because she smokes crack. Her risk is heightened as she moves through various stages of drug use and at some point may find herself trading sex for money or crack.

First, poor African-American women who eventually go on to smoke crack begin as a potential crack user observing others in the high-risk environment in different roles and carrying out different responsibilities. At this stage the woman may not be a crack user herself. She may drink or smoke marijuana but has not graduated to the stigmatized crack cocaine. As she uses these other "gateway" drugs, she is able to observe the crack culture because she most likely is smoking marijuana and drinking alcohol in the same high-risk environment. Yet she has not crossed the line to learn how to use the tools for smoking crack. Generally, someone offers it to her. She may refuse on the first offer, as she cannot see herself taking part in the crack subculture. However, every crack user obviously has that initial socialization moment where she is invited or elects to try crack for the first time.

No matter the initiation process, once she has smoked crack cocaine a few times, within the crack subculture, she moves from the observation stage and into the participation stage, where she has taken on a particular role as a crack user. As a newcomer to the crack culture, she may not know all the different roles and rules. She may find herself getting cheated out of money and drugs by more experienced users and dealers who exploit her status as newcomer. As she interacts more with others in the crack-using scene, she becomes familiar with more of the roles and responsibilities associated with everyday living as a crack user. So, as a particular woman increases her interaction with drug users, drug dealers, and women who trade sex, she may find herself taking on some aspects of these roles in the play stage. If she interacts more with drug dealers, she may attempt to sell drugs for someone rather than become a sex worker to supply her habit. In any case, during this second stage, a drug user begins to distinguish between a number of social roles in the high-risk environment and spends time actively playing a role or roles. To be clear, she is probably gravitating toward a particular role that best meets her personality and other character traits.

Finally, crack users enter a third stage where they learn more about the elaborate rules and roles of the drug culture. Poor African-American women who advance to this stage may be harder to reach with HIV prevention messages because they are so engrossed in the crack scene. For the drug culture, this stage is synonymous with the internalization of the values and expectations of the larger society and the complex interrelationships between roles. When drug users enter this stage, much of their daily activity is governed by high-risk rules of behavior. As such, a crack user not only learns her role, but also the roles of every other player and their relationships to one another in particular situations. To paraphrase Mead (1934) in *Mind, Self, and Society*, each individual's action is determined to some extent by what she assumes other players' actions will be.

HIV risk reduction programs that target crack users must be mindful of where the at-risk person stands in the stages of socialization into the drug culture. If she is in the early stage and perhaps still has some ties to mainstream society, the intervention will have a different impact than if she has been using crack for ten or more years. For example, crack-using women who have maintained the role of "mother," "employee," or "caregiver" may have a more positive and immediate change of behavior compared to women who have little to no social support network outside the drug-using community.

There are at least two distinct extremes of reaction to HIV intervention for long-term crack users. Some may view it as a defining moment that helped them make the decision to make some positive behavioral changes. Others, however, may not attempt to make changes because they perceive those with whom they interact in the drug culture as key to their survival. In addition, one is more likely to adhere to risk reduction principles if she is at a point where it is becoming more painful and difficult to maintain the role of crack user.

RETHINKING THE HIP INTERVENTION

The HIP intervention was developed and implemented based on gender and power theory. In planning for the next generation of HIV prevention for high risk black women, we need to advance the theoretical paradigm to include key tenets of black feminism In this section I discuss some practical ways to build upon the HIP intervention in ways that can be applied to other existing women-centered HIV programs grounded in gender and power theory. Collins (2000) asserts that black feminist thought is a black woman's interpretation and explanation of social phenomenon based on the idea that we think differently about social issues. In addition, we ask different questions about the nature and solutions of social problems in comparison to our white and male counterparts. While this thought process is meant to reflect an insider's standpoint, it is by no means critical of the HIP intervention, as the women themselves have validated the effectiveness of the process by which the HIP intervention reduced their risk for HIV. I suspect they found it to be effective because it was grounded in general feminist perspectives, and thus has some commonalties with black feminism. To demonstrate this, in Table 9.1, I highlight how the five themes commonly discussed in a black feminist perspective were

TABLE 9.1. A comparison of the HIP intervention and black feminist perspective.

Theme	HIP intervention	Black feminist perspective	Implications for future interventions
Self-definition and self-valuation	Influenced by "either/or" perspectives seeking to quantify change, and is generally based on existing indicators for changed behavior	Influenced by the idea that black women judge their behavior by comparing themselves to black women facing similar situations, with change generally seen as relative to others in their environment	Develop a formal role for successful program graduates to serve as peer leaders, with a greater emphasis on culturally and gender appropriate indicators of change
Race, class, and gender	Emphasis on poor women with race underexplored	Emphasis on black women with class underexplored	Place more emphasis on understanding the social construction of race, class, and gender in each woman's life
Unique (historical experiences)	Focuses on oppression, consciousness, and action centered on the motto "The personal is political"	Historical oppression, hidden consciousness, collective action centered on the motto "Lift as we climb"	Formal programmatic ties to black churches and women civic organizations and train women as "sister advocates"
Controlling images	Replaces crackhead and crack whore images with a nonjudgmental tone toward women as sex worker and drug user	Replaces crackhead and crack whore images with positive roles for black women as mother, worker, caretaker, wife, volunteer, daughter	Develop a formal method for assisting women with reunification with family of origin and procreation, as well as job training, parenting skills, relationship counseling, and volunteer opportunities
Structure and agency	A greater emphasis on agency "Here is a list of services and agencies. Let me know how it goes"	A greater balance between structure constraints and self-empowerment "Here's an advocate who will help you access services and navigate through the intensity and politics associated with assessment and in-take processes for community-based programs"	Formally train community-based organizations as mentors/advocates that increase links to services

addressed in the HIP project. In addition, I show how black feminism is different in scope in comparison to general feminist approaches to action research. As these observations arise from the women in this study, they represent what Lorde (1996) calls an "authentic black feminist standpoint" because the perspectives are from those experiencing the problems first hand.

In examining the theme of self-definition, the HIP project used quantitative methods to determine if women changed their risky behavior. Black feminism questions "either/or thinking" because it forces black women to choose between extremes when their true experiences might fall along a continuum. In addition, a black feminist perspective acknowledges that black women define their success or failure based on other black women facing the same situation as being the norm. In this case, then, the HIP project could have enhanced its effectiveness among black women by using successful program graduates as peer leaders and finding a formal role for them in the prevention intervention program. Perhaps such an approach would have been beneficial for the "hard to reach and retain."

Next, in terms of intersecting oppressions, the HIP project related to the women's class and gender status—as poor women—and may have left race somewhat underexplored. At the same time, one of the weaknesses of black feminism is that it speaks of including all women but tends to privilege black middle- and upper-class women. Thus, a future program would be effective in formalizing a process by which the women could provide richer details on how they grapple with the intersection of race, class, and gender.

In addressing the women's unique experiences, the HIP model was geared more toward the feminist motto "the personal is political," implying a greater emphasis on self-empowerment in order to change one's circumstances. The historical motto of black women has been "lift as we climb," indicating that as a sisterhood fighting multiple oppressions, black women must model the change behavior they seek in others. The practical enhancement for the HIP model would be formal group discussions with women who are tied to the church and community, where this motto originated. As the sessions at the HIP House were individual in nature, it may have left a historically effective change process for black women underutilized. My recommendation of formal group discussions is not to be confused with group discussion limited to women who use drugs.

Specifically, the women expressed needing help with housing, escaping domestic violence, regaining custody of or visitation with children, and other legal issues generally associated with drug law violations. Others wanted social support while in drug treatment, help with job hunting, and transportation to various community-based resources. Another group expressed a desire to have help in establishing communication with their extended family and children. These are all ways in which non–drug-using women committed to "lift as they climb" could help enhance interventions for the socially isolated.

I believe the HIP intervention was quite effective in helping women have dignity even on the margins. I saw women walk into intervention rooms with lowered heads and tearful eyes. Many would walk out an hour later with a smile and chin up. I believe this was due to the way each interventionist facilitated discussions about the women's roles as drug users and sex workers in a noncondemning environment. However, as the process interviews revealed, the women would like to have talked more about themselves in other roles, as mentioned in Table 9.1, whether present or past. A black feminist perspective challenges the women to set goals based on the roles and images they would like to have in the future. As many women expressed wanting a better relationship with their mothers and children in particular, another enhancement would be a formal role for the women's biological family in risk reduction. Again, this thought stems from the historical role that black mothers have played in their children's lives.

Finally, the theme of structure and agency was present in the HIP intervention. For example, if a woman received an enhanced session, then her interventionist could help her access community and social services. I argue that the intervention placed more emphasis on agency, as interventionists often provided a list of services and had no formal system for assisting women. To be clear, many interventionists maintained contact with some women well beyond their ties to the HIP intervention. However, a black feminist approach would recognize that women on the margins need systematic help in navigating through the politics associated with getting social resources. As such, advocacy should take on a more formal role in HIV intervention.

The significance of black feminist thought in HIV prevention intervention is its acknowledgement that African-American women have agency, and even in dire poverty, a sense of empowerment to think and act toward changing their own oppressive situations (Taylor, 1998). The women in this study have defined themselves as capable of making long-term changes if they have the right environment and mindset. As these women articulated their struggles within the context of their living arrangements, the solutions to their problems should take into account improved housing. I have attempted to outline what a black feminist approach to intervention might look like in the lives of African-American women at risk as grounded in the five major themes Collins argues represent black feminist perspective. Clearly, my suggestions are meant to enhance the effectiveness of the HIP intervention as a way to capture those women (1) who did not make changes in their sex or drug-using behaviors; (2) who made short-term changes and reverted back to risk behavior in three months or less; and (3) who were ready to make changes just as their HIP intervention was ending.

AN HIV PREVENTION MODEL FOR BLACK WOMEN GUIDED BY BLACK FEMINISM

Black feminist theory posits that HIV prevention intervention programs address unique issues in the lives of poor African-American women. Helping African-American women to become more empowered merely begins the risk reduction process. Risk reduction must include the transformation of unjust social institutions that African-American women encounter from one generation to the next. Black feminist perspective can contribute to a paradigm shift in how HIV prevention interventionists think about the unjust power relations that shape black women's risk for HIV. By embracing a paradigm of intersecting oppressions of race, class, and gender to critique structural domains of power, black feminist thought reconceptualizes the social relations of domination and resistance (Collins, 1990).

Given the continued increase in the number of new cases of HIV/ AIDS among poor African-American women who use crack cocaine, we know that a simple transfer of risk reduction strategies is not the most effective method for reversing the trend among this high-risk group. For the most part, public health scholars and practitioners have ignored African-American women's unique history when designing and implementing risk reduction. A careful examination and appreciation for African-American women's socialization in the United States would provide historical evidence as to how this group survives and resists harm (Gray-White, 1999; White, 1994).

New theories for HIV prevention should arise from among the new faces and factors that are disproportionately impacted by HIV (De-Carlo and Kelly, 1996). By incorporating key components of black feminist theory into existing HIV preventions, researchers can take a closer look at what works in the lives of poor African-American women who smoke crack, when designing more effective programs. Perhaps, black feminists' most radical premise has been their rejection not only of what is concluded about black women, "but the credibility and the intentions of those possessing the power to define" (Collins, 1991a). According to Collins, when black women define themselves, they clearly reject the assumption that those in positions granting them the authority to describe and analyze reality are entitled to do so.

The acronym that serves as a black feminist model for HIV risk reduction is entitled "CURES," with each letter representing a key theme in black feminism (Table 9.2). In addition, for each theme, I have developed a module objective as well as some suggested activities that HIV prevention-focused community-based organizations can use to enhance their currently funded programs. HIV prevention program coordinators can work closely with local professors in women's studies, African-American studies, or sociology departments who have expertise in black feminist theory to gain technical assistance in leading suggested discussions and activities.

In conclusion, an analysis of how women came to be at risk for HIV in the first place is at the heart of black feminist thought as critical theory. Existing public health theories can address in general that "something is wrong" in these women's lives. However, black feminism explains high-risk black women's dilemma from a race, class, and gender perspective in a way that helps interventionists toward a culturally relevant approach to risk reduction. Black feminism argues that change management should reflect the women's definition of what exactly is wrong, including the women's accounts of how they be-

TABLE 9.2. CURES: A behaviorial change module based on black feminism.

Black feminist theme	Module objective	Suggested activities
C Controlling images	To help black women and HIV prevention counselors understand how controlling images are designed to make racism, sexism, poverty, and other forms of injustice appear to be natural, normal, and inevitable parts of everyday life	Discuss and process how specific controlling images constructed for black women continue to threaten black women's mental and physical health
U Unique historical experiences	To help high-risk women and HIV prevention counselors examine black women's unique experiences in balancing work and family life under oppressive conditions	Discuss the process of enslavement, segregated employment, and black feminization of poverty as continued barriers in the lives of black women
R Race, class, and gender	To help high-risk women and HIV prevention counselors more effectively address the ways in which race, class, and gender inequalities intersect in the lives of poor black women at risk for HIV	Explore what it means to be a poor black woman in the era of welfare reform and dismantling of public housing at a time when crack cocaine and HIV infection continue to disproportionately impact black women
E Expressions of self-definition and self-valuation	To help high-risk women and HIV prevention counselors appropriately apply the transtheoretical stages of change in the lives of high-risk black women	Discuss women in the various stages of change within the context of being a high-risk black woman: precontemplation; contemplation; ready for action; action; maintenance; and relapse
S Structure and agency	To help high-risk women and HIV prevention counselors bridge the gap between individual responsibility for HIV prevention and structural barriers	Promote economic empowerment by sponsoring intense job skills building and workplace etiquette; create volunteer experiences for Developing a Sister Advocacy Program to serve as an adult mentoring program; conduct a Graduation Ceremony to serve as an indicator of women's capability for completing risk reduction programs

came drug users, and how this behavior relates to their risk for HIV infection. In addition, black feminist scholars are adamant that researchers address race, class, and gender inequalities that impact poor African-American women's ability to make permanent changes.

HIV prevention programs in the lives of poor African-American women who smoke crack tend to focus on the individuals, while failing to confront institutionalized oppression. Even when such interventions claim to be culturally relevant in addressing these women's issues, they often emphasize internalized oppression, rather than structural oppression. Black feminist thought challenges both personal and institutional malfunctions as barriers to successful risk reduction. While it is critical that each woman examines her own experiences in the context of larger societal systems of domination, she may be ill-equipped to do so in the short term. It is in this context that I, as an African-American woman within the HIV prevention community, can help in interpreting the macroissues of racism, sexism, and poverty in relation to high-risk behaviors.

Although I have never used crack cocaine, been homeless, been beaten, or been pregnant, these are still issues that impact my life as a woman of color. As Dr. King so eloquently put it, "we are caught in an inescapable network of mutuality, tied in a single garment of destiny. Whatever affects one of us directly, affects all indirectly." Thus, in realizing that my liberation remains tied to the poorest among my race and gender, I do not conclude in this book; rather, I commit to clinical research and activism that results in the elimination of health disparities. As articulated throughout this book, HIV prevention in the future will need to address both individual and institutional change. Public health strategies for HIV prevention will be more effective if they integrate black feminism into the design, implementation, evaluation, and activist stages of HIV programs. The women's stories help toward such new approaches by clarifying structure and agency in their lives as it relates to HIV infection and crack cocaine use. It is their voice about their lived experiences and best strategies for changing their behavior that should be the loudest in developing the next generation of HIV prevention aimed at addressing the unique and devastating toll this disease has taken in the lives of black women.

References

Amaro, H. (1995). "Love, Sex, Power: Considering Women's Realities in HIV Prevention." *American Psychologist* 50: 437-447.

Amaro, H., and A. Raj. (2000). "On the Margin: Power and Women's HIV Risk Reduction Strategies." *Sex Roles* 42: 723-749.

Anderson, E. (1990). *Street Wise: Race, Class, and Change in an Urban Community.* Chicago, IL: University of Chicago Press.

————. (1999). *Code of the Street.* New York: W. W. Norton.

Archie-Booker, D., R. Cervero, and C. Langone. (1999). "The Politics of Planning Culturally Relevant AIDS Prevention Education for African-American Women." *Adult Education Quarterly* 46(4): 163-170.

Auerback, J. D., and T. J. Coates. (2000). "HIV Prevention Research: Accomplishments and Challenges for the Third Decade of AIDS." *American Journal of Public Health* 90(7): 1029-1032.

Bach, V., and S. Y. West. (1993). *Housing on the Block: Divestment and Abandonment Risks in New York City Neighborhoods.* New York: Community Service Society of New York.

Bandura, A. (1994). "Social Cognitive Theory and Exercise of Control over HIV Infection." In *Preventing AIDS: Theories and Methods of Behavioral Interventions,* edited by R. DiClemente and J. Peterson (pp. 25-59). New York: Plenum Press.

Bartelt, D. (1993). "Housing the 'Underclass'" In *The "Underclass" Debate: Views from History,* edited by M. B. Katz (pp. 118-57). Princeton, NJ: Princeton University Press.

Battle, R. S., G. L. Cummings, J. C. Barker, and F. M. Krasnovsky. (1995). "Accessing an Understudied Population in Behavioral HIV/AIDS Research: Low Income African American Women." *Journal of Health and Social Policy* 7(2): 1-18.

Battle, R. S., G. L. Cummings, K. A. Yamada, and F. M. Krasnovsky. (1996). "HIV Testing Among Low-Income African-American Mothers." *AIDS Education and Prevention* 8(2): 165-175.

Benokraitis, N. V. (1999). *Marriages and Families: Changes, Choices, and Constraints.* Upper Saddle River, NJ: Prentice Hall.

Berg, B. (2001). *Qualitative Research Methods for the Social Sciences.* Boston: Allyn and Bacon.

Berger, P. L., and T. Luckmann. (1966). *The Social Construction of Reality: A Treatise Its the Sociology of Knowledge.* Garden City, NY: Anchor Books.

Black Women's Risk for HIV: Rough Living
© 2007 by The Haworth Press, Taylor & Francis Group. All rights reserved.
doi:10.1300/5784_10   *249*

Blankenship, K. M., S. J. Bray, and M. H. Merson. (2000). "Structural Interventions in Public Health." *AIDS* 14: S11-S21.

Blumer, H. (1969). *Symbolic Interactionism: Perspective and Method*. Englewood Cliffs, NJ: Prentice Hall.

Bourgois, P. (1995). *In Search of Respect: Selling Crack in El Barrio*. Cambridge, MA: University Press.

Bowleg, L., F. Z. Belgrave, and C. A. Reisen. (2000). "Gender Roles, Power Strategies, and Precautionary Sexual Self-Efficacy: Implications for Black and Latina Women's HIV/AIDS Protective Behaviors." *Sex Roles* 42(7): 613-635.

Boyd, C. J. (1993). "The Antecedents of Women's Crack Cocaine Abuse: Family Substance Abuse, Sexual Abuse, Depression and Illicit Drug Use." *Journal of Substance Abuse Treatment* 10: 433-438.

Boyle, K., and M. D. Anglin. (1993). "To the Curb: Sex Bartering and Drug Use Among Homeless Crack Users in Los Angeles." In *Crack Pipe as Pimp: An Ethnographic Investigation of Sex-for-Crack Exchanges*, edited by M. S. Ratner (pp. 159-85). New York: Lexington Books.

Centers for Disease Control and Prevention. (2001). *Surveillance Report*. Atlanta, GA: CDC Division of HIV/AIDS.

Centers for Disease Control and Prevention. (2006). *HIV/AIDS Surveillance Report, 2005*. Vol. 17. Atlanta: US Department of Health and Human Services, CDC, pp. 1-46.

Collins, P. H. (1991a). "Learning from the Outsider Within: The Social Significance of Black Feminist Thought." In *Beyond Methodology*, edited by M. Fonow and J. Cook (pp. 35-59). Bloomington: Indiana University Press.

———. (1991b). "The Meaning of Motherhood in Black Culture." In *The Black Family: Essays and Studies*, edited by R. Staples (pp. 157-166). Belmont, CA: Wadsworth.

———. (1998). *Fighting Words: Black Women and the Search for Justice*. Minneapolis: University of Minnesota Press.

———. (2000). *Black Feminist Thought: Knowledge, Consciousness, and the Politics of Empowerment*, second edition. New York: Routledge Press.

Comfort, M., O. A. Grinstead, B. Faigeles, and B. Zack. (2000). "Reducing HIV Risk Among Women Visiting Their Incarcerated Male Partners." *Criminal Justice and Behavior* 27(1): 57-71.

Cooley, C. H. (1902). *Human Nature and Social Order*. New York: Scribner's.

Crane, J., K. Quirk, and A. van der Straten. (2002). "'Come Back When You're Dying': The Commodification of AIDS Among California's Urban Poor." *Social Science Medicine* 55(7): 1115-1127.

Cummings, S. (1998). *Left Behind in Rosedale: Race Relations and the Collapse of Community Institutions*. Boulder, CO: Westview Press.

Dalla, R. (2004). "'I Fell Off [the Mothering] Track': Barriers to 'Effective Mothering' Among Prostituted Women." *Family Relations* 53: 190-200.

Dancy, B. L., R. Marcantonio, and K. Norr. (2000). "The Long-Term Effectiveness of an HIV Prevention Intervention for Low-Income African American Women." *AIDS Education and Prevention* 4(2): 113.

Dash, L. (1996). *Rosa Lee: A Mother and Her Family in Urban America*. New York: Plume.

DeCarlo, P., and J. Kelly. (1996). "Can HIV Prevention Programs Be Adapted?" *Center for AIDS Prevention Studies: AIDS Research Institute*. Retrieved April 27, 2001 from http://www.caps.ucsf.edu/capsweb/adaptext.html.

DeCarlo, P., and K. Quirk. (1998). "What Are Women's HIV Prevention Needs?" *Center for AIDS Prevention Studies: AIDS Research Institute*. Retrieved April 27, 2001 from http://www.caps.ucsf.edu/capsweb/adaptext.html.

Dittus, P., K. S. Miller, B. A. Kotchick, and R. Forehand. (2004). "Why Parents Matter! The Conceptual Basis for a Community-Based HIV Prevention Program for the Parents of African American Youth." *Journal of Child and Family Studies* 13: 5-20.

Downing, M., K. R. Knight, K. A. Vernon, S. Seigel, I. Ajaniku, P. S. Acosta, L. Thomas, and S. Porter. (1999). "This Is My Story: A Descriptive Analysis of a Peer Education HIV/STD Risk Reduction Program for Women Living in Housing Developments." *AIDS Education and Prevention* 11(3): 243-261.

Edin, K., and L. Lein. (1997). Making Ends Meet: How Single Mothers Survive Welfare and Low-Wage Work. New York: Russell Sage Foundation.

Eicher-Catt, D. (2004). "Noncustodial Mothering: A Cultural Paradox of Competent Performance: Performative Competence." *Journal of Contemporary Ethnography* 33(1): 72-108.

El-Bassel, N., S. Witte, L. Gilbert, M. Sormanti, C. Moreno, L. Pereira, E. Elam, and P. Steinglass. (2001). "HIV Prevention for Intimate Couples: A Relationship-Based Model." *Families, Systems, and Health* 19(4): 379-395.

Fagan, J. (1993). "Drug Selling and Licit Income in Distressed Neighborhoods: The Economic Lives of Street-Level Drug Users and Dealers." In *Drugs, Crime and Social Isolation*, edited by G. Peterson and A. Harrell (pp. 519-35). Washington, DC: Urban Institute Press.

Fagan, J., and K. L. Chin. (1989). "Initiation into Crack and Cocaine: A Tale of Two Epidemics." *Contemporary Drug Problems* 16: 579-617.

Fine, M., and L. Weis. (1998). *The Unknown City: Lives of Poor and Working Class Young Adults*. Boston, MA: Beacon Press.

Fisher, J., and W. A. Fisher. (2000). "Theoretical Approaches to Individual-Level Change in HIV Risk Behavior." In *Handbook of HIV Prevention*, edited by J. L. Peterson and R. DiClemente (pp. 3-35). New York: Plenum Press.

Fullilove, M., R. Fullilove, B. Bower, R. Haynes, and S. Gross. (1990). "Black Women and AIDS Prevention: A View Towards Understanding Gender Rules." *Journal of Sex Research* 27: 47-64.

Fullilove, M., R. Fullilove, M. Smith, K. Winkler, C. Michael, P. Panzer and R. Wallace. (1993). "Violence, Trauma, and Post-Traumatic Stress Disorder Among Women Drug Users." *Journal of Traumatic Stress* 6: 533-543.

Fullilove, M., E. Lown, and R. Fullilove. (1992). "Crack 'Hos and Skeezers: Traumatic Experiences of Women Crack Users." *Journal of Sex Research* 29(2): 275-287.

Gans, H. (1994). "Positive Functions of the Undeserving Poor." *Politics and Society* 22(3): 269-283.

Gentry, Q. (2004). "A Black Feminist Critique of the Social Construction of Crack Cocaine Along Race, Class, and Gender Lines." In *Race and Ethnicity: Across Time, Space and Discipline*, edited by R. D. Coates (pp. 239-253). The Netherlands: Brill Academic Publishers.

Gentry, Q. M., K. Elifson, and C. Sterk. (2005). "Aiming for More Relevant HIV Risk Reduction: A Black Feminist Perspective for Enhancing HIV Intervention for Low-Income African American Women." *AIDS Education and Prevention* 17(3): 238-252.

Geronimus, A. (2000). "To Mitigate, Resist, or Undo: Addressing Structural Influences on the Health of Urban Populations." *American Journal of Public Health* 90(6): 867-872.

Gilbert, D. J. (2003a). "Focus on Solutions: Black Churches Respond to AIDS: Interview with Pernessa C. Seele, Founder and CEO of The Balm in Gilead." In *African American Women and HIV/AIDS: Critical Responses,* edited by D. J. Gilbert and E. M. Wright (pp. 153-158). Westport, CT: Praeger.

Gilbert, D. J. (2003b). "The Sociocultural Construction of AIDS Among African American Women." In *African American Women and HIV/AIDS: Critical Responses,* edited by D. J. Gilbert and E. M. Wright (pp. 5-27). Westport, CT: Praeger.

Gilbert, D. J., and E. M. Wright. (2003). "Reconstructing the Reality of African American Women and HIV/AIDS." In *African American Women and HIV/AIDS: Critical Responses,* edited by D. J. Gilbert and E. M. Wright (pp. 1-3). Westport, CT: Praeger.

Goffman, E. (1959). *The Presentation of Self in Everyday Life.* New York: Doubleday.

Gomez, C., and B. Marin. (1996). "Gender, Culture, and Power: Barriers to HIV-Prevention Strategies for Women." *The Journal of Sex Research* 33: 355-362.

Gray-White, D. (1999). *Too Heavy a Load: Black Women in Defense of Themselves, 1894-1994.* New York: W. W. Norton.

Grinstead, O., B. Zack, and B. Faigeles. (1999). "Collaborative Research to Prevent HIV Among Male Prison Inmates and Their Female Partners." *Health Education and Behavior* 26(2): 225-238.

Guy-Sheftall, B. (1995). Words of Fire: An Anthology of African-American Feminist Thought. New York: New Press.

Hardesty, M., and T. Black. (1999). "Mothering Through Addiction: A Survival Strategy Among Puerto Rican Addicts." *Qualitative Health Research* 9(5): 602-619.

Harlow, L., J. S. Rose, P. J. Morokoff, K. Quina, K. Mayer, K. Mitchell, and R. Schnoll. (1998). "Women HIV Sexual Risk Takers: Related Behaviors, Interpersonal Issues, and Attitudes." *Women's Health* 4(4): 407-39.

Hays, S. (1996). *The Cultural Contradictions of Motherhood.* New Haven, CT: Yale University Press.

The Holy Bible, King James Version (KJV). (1979). Nashville, TN: Thomas Nelson, Inc. Publishers.

Holzier, H. (1995). *What Employers Want: Job Prospects for Less-Educated Workers.* New York: Russell Sage Foundation.

hooks, b. (1981). *Ain't I a Woman: Black Women and Feminism*. Boston: South End Press.
———. (1984). *Feminist Theory: From Margin to Center*. Boston: South End Press.
Jackson, R. (1994). *Mothers Who Leave: Behind the Myth of Women Without Their Children*. London: Pandora.
Jackson, R., and B. Reddick. (1999). "The African American Church and University Partnerships: Establishing Lasting Collaborations." *Health Education and Behavior* 26(5): 663-674.
James, W. (1890). *The Principles of Psychology*. New York: Henry Holt.
Kadushin, G. (1996). "Gay Men with AIDS and Their Families of Origin: An Analysis of Social Support." *Health and Social Work* 21(2): 141-149.
Kalichman, S., E. Williams, C. Charsey, L. Belcher, and D. Nachimson. (1998). "Sexual Coercion, Domestic Violence, and Negotiating Condom Use Among Low-Income African American Women." *Journal of Women's Health* 7(3): 371-379.
Kane, S., and T. Mason. (1992). "'IV Drug Users' and 'Sex Partners': The Limits of Epidemiological Categories and the Ethnography of Risk." In *The Time of AIDS: Social Analysis, Theory, and Methods,* edited by G. Herdt and S. Lindenbaum (pp. 199-222). Newbury Park, CA: Sage.
Kearney, M., S. Murphy, and M. Rosenbaum. (1994). "Mothering on Crack Cocaine: A Grounded Theory Analysis." *Social Science Medicine* 38: 351-361.
Kelly, E. (2003). "African American Adolescent Girls: Neglected and Disrespected." In *African American Women and HIV/AIDS: Critical Responses,* edited by D. J. Gilbert and E. M. Wright (pp. 163-182). Westport, CT: Praeger.
King, D. (1988). "Multiple Jeopardy, Multiple Consciousness: The Context of a Black Feminist Ideology." *Signs* 14: 42-72.
Kirschenman, J., and K. Neckerman. (1991). "'We'd Love to Hire Them, But . . .': The Meaning of Race for Employers." In *The Urban Underclass,* edited by C. Jencks and P. Peterson (pp. 203-234). Washington, DC: Brookings Institution.
Kline, A., E. Kline, and E. Oken. (1992). "Minority Women and Sexual Choices in the Age of AIDS." *Social Science Medicine* 34(4): 447-457.
Ladwig, G., and M. Andersen. (1989). "Substance Abuse in Women: Relationship Between Chemical Dependency of Women and Past Reports of Physical and/or Sexual Abuse." *International Journal of the Addictions* 24: 739-754.
LaRossa, R., and D. Reitzes. (1994). "Symbolic Interactionism and Family Studies." In *Sourcebook of Family Theories and Methods: A Contextual Approach,* edited by P. G. Boss, W. J. Doherty, R. LaRossa, W. R. Schumm, and S. K. Steinmetz (pp. 135-163). New York: Plenum Press.
Lieb, J., and C. Sterk-Elifson. (1995). "Crack in the Cradle: Social Policy and Reproductive Rights Among Crack-Using Females." *Journal of Contemporary Drug Problems* 22(4): 687-705.
Liebow, E. (1993). *Tell Them Who I Am: The Lives of Homeless Women*. New York: Free Press.
Lorde, A. (1996). *Sister Outsider: Essays and Speeches*. Freedom, CA: Crossing Press.

MacCleod, J. (1995). *Ain't No Making It: Aspirations and Attainments in a Low-Income Neighborhood*, second edition. Boulder, CO: Westview Press.

Maher, L. (1990). "Criminalizing Pregnancy: The Downside of a Kinder Gentler Nation." *Criminal Justice* 17: 111-135.

Maines, D. (1989). "Herbert Blumer and the Possibility of Science in the Practice of Sociology: Further Thoughts." *Journal of Contemporary Ethnography* 18: 160-177.

Massey, D., and N. Denton. (1993). *American Apartheid: Segregation and the Making of the Underclass*. Cambridge, MA: Harvard University Press.

Mead, G. (1934). *Mind, Self, and Society*. Vol. 1. Edited by C. Morris. Chicago: University of Chicago Press.

Misovich, S., J. Fisher, and W. Fisher. (1997). "Close Relationships and Elevated HIV Risk Behavior: Evidence and Possible Underlying Psychological Processes." *Review of General Psychology* 1: 72-107.

Molina, L. D., and C. Basinait-Smith. (1998). "Revisiting the Intersection Between Domestic Abuse and HIV Risk." *American Journal of Public Health* 88: 1267-1268.

Moore, J., J. S. Harrison, and L. S. Doll. (1994). "Interventions for Sexually Active, Heterosexual Women in the United States." In *Preventing AIDS: Theories and Methods of Behavioral Interventions*, edited by R. DiClemente and J. Peterson (pp. 243-265). New York: Plenum Press.

Newman, K. (1999). *No Shame in My Game*. New York: Knopf and the Russell Sage Foundation.

Nyamathi, A., and J. Stein. (1997). "Assessing the Impact of HIV Risk Reduction Counseling in Impoverished African American Women: A Structural Equations Approach." *AIDS Education and Prevention* 9(3): 254-273.

O'Leary, A., and P. Martin. (2000). "Structural Factors Affecting Women's HIV Risk: A Life Course Example." *AIDS* 14: S68-S72.

O'Leary, A., and G. Wingood. (2000). "Intervention for Sexually Active Heterosexual Women." Pp. 179-200 in *Handbook of HIV Prevention*, edited by J. Peterson and R. DiClemente. New York: Plenum Press.

Patton, M. (1990). *Qualitative Evaluation and Research Methods*. Newbury Park, CA: Sage.

Pulerwitz, J., S. L. Gortmaker, and DeJong, W. (2000). "Measuring Sexual Relationship Power in HIV/STD Research." *Sex Roles* 42(7/8): 637-660.

Quina, K., L. L. Harlow, P. J. Morokoff, G. Burkholder, and P. J. Deiter. (2000). "Sexual Communication in Relationships: When Words Speak Louder than Actions." *Sex Roles* 42(7/8): 523-549.

Reeves, P. M., S. B. Merriam, and B. C. Courtenay. (1999). "Adaptation to HIV Infection: The Development of Coping Strategies Over Time." *Qualitative Health Research* 9(3): 344-361.

Roberts, C. (1999). "Drug Use Among Inner-City African American Women: The Process of Managing Loss." *Qualitative Health Research* 9(5): 620-638.

Roberts, D. (1991). "Punishing Drug Addicts Who Have Babies: Women of Color, Equality, and the Right of Privacy." *Harvard Law Review* 194: 1419-1482.

———. (1997). *Killing the Black Body*. New York: Vintage Books.

Scott, K., A. Gilliam, and K. Braxton. (2005). "Culturally Competent HIV Prevention Strategies for Women of Color in the United States." *Health Care for Women International* 26: 17-45.

Sharpe, T. T. (2001). "Sex-for-Crack-Cocaine Exchange, Poor Black Women, and Pregnancy." *Qualitative Health Research* 11(5): 612-630.

Sherman, S., A. Gielen, and K. McDonnell. (2000). "Power and Attitudes in Relationships (PAIR) Among a Sample of Low-Income, African-American Women: Implications for HIV/AIDS Prevention." *Sex Roles* 41(3/4): 283-294.

Sobo, E. (1995). *Choosing Unsafe Sex: AIDS-Risk Denial Among Disadvantaged Women*. Philadelphia: University of Pennsylvania Press.

Sterk, C. (1999). *Fast Lives: Women Who Use Crack Cocaine*. Philadelphia: Temple University Press.

Sterk, C., and K. Elifson. (2003). "A Qualitative Case Study." In *Community-Based Research: Issues and Methods*, edited by D. Blumenthal and R. DiClemente (pp. 153-170). New York: Springer.

Sterk, C., K. Elifson, and D. German. (2000). "Female Crack Users and Their Sexual Relationships: The Role of Sex-for-Crack Exchanges." *The Journal of Sex Research* 37(4): 354-360.

Sterk-Elifson, C., and K. Elifson. (1993). "The Social Organization of Crack Cocaine Use: The Cycle in One Type of Base House." *Journal of Drug Issues* 23: 429-441.

Stryker, S. (1980). *Symbolic Interactionism*. Menlo Park, CA: Sage.

Sumartojo, E. (2000). "Structural Factors in HIV Prevention: Concepts, Examples, and Implications for Research." *AIDS* 14(1): S3-S10.

Sylvia, P. (2001). *Where We Draw the Line: The Allocation of Amenities Within Four Neighborhoods in and Around Atlanta*. Master's thesis, Georgia State University.

Taylor, U. (1998). "Making Waves: The Theory and Practice of Black Feminism." *The Black Scholar* 28(2): 18-28.

Thomas, W. (1972). "The Definition of the Situation." In *Symbolic Interaction: A Reader in Social Psychology,* edited by J. Manis and B. Meltzer (pp. 331-336). Boston: Allyn and Bacon.

Thurer, S. (1994). *The Myths of Motherhood: How Culture Reinvents the Good Mother*. Boston: Houghton Mifflin.

Tross, S. (2001). "Women at Heterosexual Risk for HIV in Inner-City New York: Reaching the Hard to Reach." *AIDS and Behavior* 5(2): 131-139.

U.S. Bureau of the Census. (1990). "Characteristics of the Population." Summary Tape File 3. Washington, DC: U.S. Census Bureau. Retrieved April 20, 2001 from http://venus.census.gov/cdrom/lookup/.

U.S. Census Bureau. (2000). "Thematic Map Frames." Summary File 1 (SF 1) and Summary File 3 (SF 3). Washington, DC: U.S. Census Bureau. Retrieved May 7, 2007 from http://factfinder.census.gov/servlet/ThematicMapFramesetServlet.

Vogt, E., and M. A. Leeper. (2000). "HIV/AIDS Prevention Messages Elude African American Women." *Healthcare PR and Marketing News* 9: 17.

Wallace, B. (1990). "Crack Cocaine Smokers as Adult Children of Alcoholics: The Dysfunctional Family Link." *Journal of Substance Abuse Treatment* 7: 89-100.

Wallace, R. (1993). "Social Disintegration and the Spread of AIDS—II. Meltdown of Sociographic Structure in Urban Minority Neighborhoods." *Social Science and Medicine* 37: 887-896.

Ward, M. (1993). "A Different Disease: HIV/AIDS and Health Care for Women in Poverty." *Culture, Medicine, and Psychiatry* 17: 298-301.

Wexler, H., S. Magura, M. Beardsley, and H. Josepher. (1994). "ARRIVE: An AIDS Education/Relapse Prevention Model for High-Risk Parolees." *International Journal of the Addictions* 29: 361-386.

White, E., ed. (1994). *The Black Women's Health Book: Speaking for Ourselves.* Seattle, WA: Seal Press.

Whyte, W. (1981). *Street Corner Society.* 3d ed. Chicago: University of Chicago Press.

Wilson, W. (1996). *When Work Disappears: The World of the New Urban Poor.* New York: Knopf.

Woods, I. (1998). "Bringing Harm Reduction to the Black Community." In *Harm Reduction,* edited by G. Alan Marlatt (pp. 301-326). New York: Guilford Press.

Worth, D. (1989). "Sexual Decision-Making and AIDS: Why Condom Promotion Among Vulnerable Women Is Likely to Fail." *Studies in Family Planning* 20: 297-307.

Index

Page numbers followed by the letter "t" indicate tables; those followed by the letter "f" indicate figures; and those followed by the letter "e" indicate exhibits.

Absolute homeless, 28, 32, 60
Abused self, 93
Action stage, 210
Anderson, Elijah, 58-59, 66
Atlanta University Center, 2

Behavioral change theory, 209
Berg, Bruce, 14
Biblical doctrine, 209
Black feminism
    behavior change theory, 233
    as critical theory, 15-16, 21, 246
    HIV prevention intervention, 60
    motherhood, 133
    poverty, 3-4
    risk and resilience, 66
    self-definition and self-valuation, 93
    structure and agency, 164, 195
    unique experiences, 97, 167
Blumer, Herbert, 17

Casual partners, 97
Centers for Disease Control and
    Prevention, xii, 4
Child welfare, 156
Chronically homeless, 188
Church, 196-197, 200
Churched women, 196
Civil Rights Movement, xii
Code of the streets, 66
Code switch, 11

Co-dependency theory, 124
Co-dependent couples, 113
Commitment stage, 99, 103, 129
A comparison of the HIP intervention
    and black feminist
    perspective, 242t
Compromise stage, 99, 115-116, 130
Concentrated poverty, 74
Concentrated unemployment, 58
Conclusion stage, 99, 120, 130
Concurrent commitments, 112
Concurrent intimate partners, 117-118
Conditions of hopeful and hopeless
    mothering, 160t
Conflict stage, 99, 112, 129
Contemplation, 209
Controlling images, 16, 150, 242, 247
Conversating to avoid dating, 177
Cooley, Charles, 17
Couple-centered HIV prevention, 112
Courtship stage, 99-101, 128
Crack babies, 135
Crack cocaine economy, 192
Critical theory, 15
CURES, 246
CURES: A behavioral change module
    based on black feminism,
    247t
Custody to kin, 140-141

Decent families, 2, 7, 59, 63, 66-67, 75
Decent or street girls, 8

Depression, 202
Desegregation, 1-2
Deserving and undeserving poor, 59
Domestic violence
    absolute homeless, 60-61
    commitment stage of relationships,
        110
    condom use, 125-126
    conflict stage of relationships, 114
    house women, 54
    indicator of risk for HIV, 83
    normal, 80-81
    pregnant, 65
Dominant gender script, 98
Dominant HIV prevention script of
        condom use, 125
Drug and sex behavior, 54
Drug treatment, 11, 146, 212, 221
Dualistic thinking, 235

Ethnographic findings, 8
Ethnographic research methods, 10

Faith-based institution, 204, 205
FAITH-model, 206
The FAITH-Model for faith-based HIV
        prevention capacity building,
        207e
Families of orientation, 76
    author's perspective, 65
    deceiving family members, 90-91
    definition, 64
    family-focused HIV prevention
        initiatives, 94-95
    family housed, 51-52
    maintaining relations, 91-92
    strengths and barriers, 84-85
Family-focused intervention, 95
Foster care system, 86, 135, 139, 157
Full-time street women, 52

Gans, Herbert, 190, 192
Gatekeepers, 11
Gender differences, 64
Gender norms, 103
Gender and power, 130

The generalized other, 239
Gentrification, 3
Ghetto poor neighborhood, 3, 9, 58, 74
Gift for gab, 177-178
Grandmothering, 136, 147
Growing up street, 77

Heads of household, 47
Heightened conflict, 113
Heterosexual HIV transmission, 4
High-risk behavior, 5-6, 8, 58, 82,
        85-86
High-risk couples, 61
High-risk environment, 2, 8, 29, 37, 58
High-risk heterosexual women, 97
High-risk sex, 30
High-risk women, 7
High-risk women's current ties to faith-
        based institutions, 205t
High-risk youth, 63-64
HIP (Health Intervention Project), 4, 7,
        9
HIP program participants
    Allison, 53-54, 63, 71, 108-109,
        114, 143-144, 182, 187, 204,
        220
    Carmen, 53, 55, 104, 184
    Corie, 47-48, 185-186, 203, 226-227
    Cynthia, 54, 69-70, 121-122
    Daisy, 68, 92, 197, 223
    Dee-Dee, 25, 29, 53, 55, 75-76, 179,
        188-189, 204
    Doll, 42-43, 76, 85, 144, 151, 196
    Dorothy, 32-33, 89, 173-174, 177,
        195, 197, 199, 214, 221
    Erica, 78-80, 102-103, 107-108,
        113, 142
    Frankie, 47, 105-106, 116, 137,
        154-155, 203
    Gayle, 64-66
    Gloria, 43, 73, 145, 187, 198
    Ingrid, 54, 112
    Janice, 35-37, 80-81, 111, 114, 117,
        141, 152-153, 173, 175-176,
        197, 212, 222
    Jennifer, 92, 120-121, 152
    Johnsie, 40-41, 76, 91, 111, 142,
        144, 155-156, 174-175,
        182-183, 185

HIP program participants *(continued)*
Ka-Ka, 106-107, 213
Karen, 47, 88, 97, 100-101,
178-180, 198, 225-226
Kawana, 159, 161-162, 172,
217-220, 224
Lisa, 47-50, 90, 123, 125, 133,
137-138, 172, 200
Lois, 53, 55-56, 139, 147-148, 155,
158-159, 177-178, 200
Lolita, 72, 227
Martha, 47-48, 109, 117, 122-123,
147, 180-182, 202-203,
215-216
Mattie, 79-80, 204
Michelle, 44-45, 52, 141, 146-147,
178
Mona, 30-32, 57, 86, 123, 156-157,
188, 201, 213-214, 222
Nicole, 6-7
Pamela, 44-46, 87, 104-105, 147,
153-154, 162-164, 199
Pauline, 75, 85, 89, 184, 203, 211,
225
Peaches, 47-48, 70-71, 118-119,
177, 181
Portia, 29-30, 68, 91, 149, 159, 202,
230
Punkin, 1-2, 4-5, 53-56, 83,
119-120, 157, 202
Sabrina, 43, 123-125, 140
Shanese, 92, 115, 142, 185
Shante, 47, 81-82, 87-88, 119, 139,
146
Sharon, 116-117, 143, 158, 172,
176, 187, 204
Sonya, 51, 87
Stephanie, 86, 167
Sunnie, 148, 186, 203, 227-228
Teresa, 41, 73, 74, 228-229,
233-234
Tomeka, 53-54, 82, 203
Tosha, 118, 145, 156
Tracie, 28, 67-68, 89-90, 223
Trina, 185
Valerie, 37-40, 142-143, 175, 215,
223-225, 230
Wanda, 86, 186-187, 199-201
Yolanda, 33-34, 171, 230-231
HIV infection, 137, 223
HIV positive, 1, 5, 87, 228

HIV prevention case manager, 201
HIV prevention intervention, 5, 7-8, 64
HIV prevention messages, 61, 121
HIV prevention program, 4, 7, 95, 128
HIV prevention research, 97
HIV risk reduction program, 201
HIV test, 15, 50
HIV/AIDS, *xi*, 2-3, 31
Homelessness, 2, 30-31, 59, 86, 110
Homeownership, 67
hooks, bell, 236
Hopeful mothers, 136, 140, 145-146,
159, 161
Hopeless mothers, 136, 148-149, 151,
159
House manager, 34, 180
House women, 46-51
Housing projects, 40, 47, 79
Hustling condoms, 179
Hustling homeless, 37, 61
Hustling knowledge, 169
Hustling knowledge of drugs, 170, 173,
175, 189
Hustling knowledge of sex, 176, 189

In-depth interviews, 13
Inner-city churches, 199
Intensive mothering, 133-134
Interest assessment, 208
Intimate partners, 97
Intimate relationships, 97-98, 121, 126

James, William, 17
Juggling multiple hustles, 189

Key stages of intimate partner
relationships, 99f
Kinship care, 142, 145, 152

Leading lady, 39
Liebow, Elliot, 40
Living arrangements, 25, 30
Local housing authority, 40
Loose behavior, 58
Lorde, Audre, 135, 243

Maintaining custody, 136
Maintenance, 210
Makeshift madams, 176
Matrix of domination, 234-235
Mead, George, 17, 241
Middle-class black families, 1, 92-93
Mind, Self, and Society, 241
Money-making skills building, 190
Motherhood, 133
Mules, 192
Multiple oppressions, 59
Multiple partners, 118

No changes in behavior, 228
Non-subsidized renters, 47
Normal mothering, 137-139, 148, 151

Odd-job hustlers, 184-186, 188
Other changes, 224

Package runners, 172
Participant observation, 10
Pastoral counseling, 199
Patriarchy, 150
Physical and sexual abuse, 71
Political economy, 59
Poverty line, 3
Poverty rate, 3
Practicing safer sex, 221
Precontemplation, 209
Prenatal care, 155, 165
Presentation of safe self, 238
Prevention intervention, 60
Private and public sex lives, 100
Product knowledge, 171
Public housing, 3-4, 79

Race, class, and gender, 16, 21, 37,
    236, 242, 246-247
Ready for action, 210
Reducing risk, 211
Reflecting back, 101
Relapse, 210
Religiosity, 195
Renting drug paraphernalia, 173

Renting spaces, 180-181
Research objectives, 22
Role conflict, 134, 140
Role strain, 140
Rooming housed, 41, 43-44, 61
Running packages, 172

Sanctification process, 198
Scapegoating, 190
Section 8, 44, 49
Self-definition and self-valuation, 16,
    21, 93, 242-243, 247
Sex trade, 180
Sex work, 182
Sex worker, 30, 32, 36, 44, 53, 167,
    170
Sexual abuse, 84, 92-93, 96
Sexual exploitation, 83
Shoplifting, 182-184
Social constructionist perspective,
    18-20, 22
Social isolation, 203
Social networks, 25
Social policies, 192
Social replacement theory, 95
Social service providers, 10
Socialization process, 84
Sociological imagination, 4
Stages of change, 209
Stages of change and biblical
    compatibility, 209-210t
Steady partners, 97
Steady-partner housed, 52-57
Street families, 58, 81
Street and house women, 26
Street outreach team, 10-11
Street women, 26-46
Structural context of poverty, 99
Structure and agency, 17, 242, 247
Subsidized renters, 47
Symbolic interactionism, 17, 22

Taken-for-granted assumption, 235
Temporary street women, 52, 54
Thomas, William, 17
Traditional case management, 201
Traditional gender lines, 104
Traditional risk reduction, 236

Unchurched women, 196, 203
Undercover family structures, 127
Unique experiences, 16, 64, 242-243,
        247
Urban ethnographies, 57
Urban renewal, 192
Urban-based churches, 195
U.S. Census Bureau, 3

Verbal and physical conflict, 115
Violent partner, 119

Wallace, Rodrick, 2
Welfare reform, 3, 47, 51, 192

Youth at risk for HIV, 66